The
LAMINITIS
ANSWER BOOK

over 200 questions answered

Remco Sikkel

© First edition 2021, Remco Sikkel
ISBN 978-94-93034-10-5
Original title: Antwoordenboek hoefbevangenheid : meer dan 200 vragen beantwoord

All rights reserved. No part of this book, either text or image may be used for any purpose other than personal use. Therefore, reproduction, modification, storage in a retrieval system or retransmission, in any form or by any means, electronic, mechanical or otherwise, for reasons other than personal use, is strictly prohibited without prior written permission of the author.

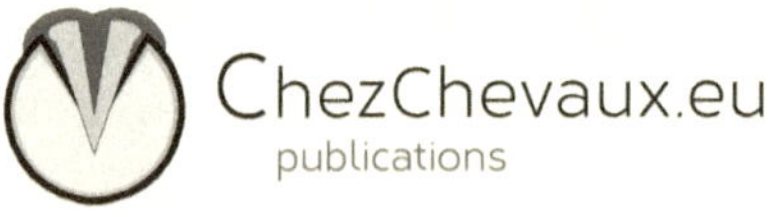

ChezChevaux.eu
publications

understandinglaminitis.com

fb.me/understandinglaminitis

From the same author: Laminitis : understanding, cure, prevention (ISBN 978-94-93034-08-2)

This book is not intended as a substitute for the medical advice of veterinarians, hoof care providers or other horse health care specialists. It just provides an overview of the current theories, diagnostic and treatment methods with regard to laminitis.
The reader should always consult a veterinarian in matters relating to their horse's health and particularly with respect to any clinical signs that may require diagnosis or medical attention. Neither the author, nor the publisher can be held accountable for any resulting damage caused by the application of the information in this book.

TABLE OF CONTENTS

CAUSES

DIAGNOSIS

TREATMENT

NUTRITION

HOUSING AND MOVEMENT

HOOF CARE

AND WHAT ABOUT ME?

FOREWORD

Your horse, pony or donkey has laminitis. It is the first time this has happened, and you are in a state of shock. Or it is the umpteenth time, and you are getting desperate. Fortunately, the Internet is bulging with information on this nasty disease. Facebook is full of good advice too. But after spending days in front of your computer screen, you feel dizzy. There are so many different ideas, opinions and advice that you can no longer see the wood for the trees. You just want clear answers to your questions. Questions like 'Do I need to soak hay? How do I do that?' and 'Could a vaccine or a worm treatment be the cause?'. You want to know whether or not you can feed willow branches to your horse. And what about therapeutic shoeing or those fancy hoof boots?

This book provides crystal-clear, practical answers to more than 200 questions about laminitis. Questions that crop up, time and again in all sorts of Facebook groups. Answers that are actually useful. This book will definitely help you and your horse.

THE HOOF

WHAT IS A HORSE HOOF?

Fifty-four million years ago, the oldest ancestor of the modern horse had five toes on each of its feet. This Eohippus was succeeded in evolution by horses with fewer and fewer toes. The splint bones that we still find in the modern horse are remnants of the 'old' toes. The Equus Caballus, our current horse, originated a million years ago. He only has one toe on each limb: the hoof. The hooves bear the full weight of the horse's body. Horses are so-called unguligrade animals. Unguligrade means 'walking on hooves'.

WHY IS HOOF HEALTH SO IMPORTANT?

Farrier and anatomist Jeremiah Bridges published a book in the mid-18th century with the legendary title, 'No foot, no horse'. The fact that we talked about horses that lived more than 50 million years ago in the previous section means that they evolved successfully. This is largely due to their hooves. Unguligrade animals can thrust very well on hard soils. This allows them to run fast when there is danger. The rigid hoof wall also protects the vulnerable inside of the hoof very effectively. A wild horse with healthy, strong hooves is more likely to survive and reproduce than a horse with poor-quality hooves.

Healthy hooves are essential for domestic horses as well. You don't want your horse to experience discomfort, pain or even lameness. In a healthy hoof, all anatomical structures are well developed and in fine-tuned balance with each other. The hoof mechanism (see p. 16) functions optimally. This ensures the entire hoof to have good blood circulation. The healthy hoof acts as a powerful shock absorber. A horse with healthy hooves will be better able to cope with any impending laminitis.

WHAT DO I NEED TO KNOW ABOUT HOW THE HOOF HAS BEEN BUILT UP TO UNDERSTAND THIS BOOK?

If we look at the hoof from the outside, we see the hoof capsule. This fits around the so-called internal foot like a shoe. The hoof capsule consists of the hoof wall, the white line, the sole, the frog and the heel bulbs. The internal foot is made up of bones, tendons and ligaments, cartilage, connective tissue, skin, blood vessels, and nerves.

The coffin bone is the lower bone in the hoof capsule. Together with the short pastern bone and the navicular bone, it forms the coffin joint (or distal interphalangeal joint). The deep digital flexor tendon runs over the navicular bone. This tendon is attached to the bottom of the coffin bone. On the other side, it is connected to the deep flexor muscle. The pull of the flexor muscle is transferred to the coffin bone through the tendon. The muscle and tendon enable the horse to flex the foot backwards. The extensor tendon connects the extensor muscle to the front of the coffin bone. This muscle and tendon enable the horse to stretch the foot forward.

The hoof cartilages (or collateral cartilages) are found at the back of the hoof and can be felt next to the bulb groove just above the level of the coronary band. At the bottom it merges into the digital cushion. This is connective tissue that acts as a shock absorber between the sole and the frog on one side and the tendons, bones, joints and hoof cartilages on the other.

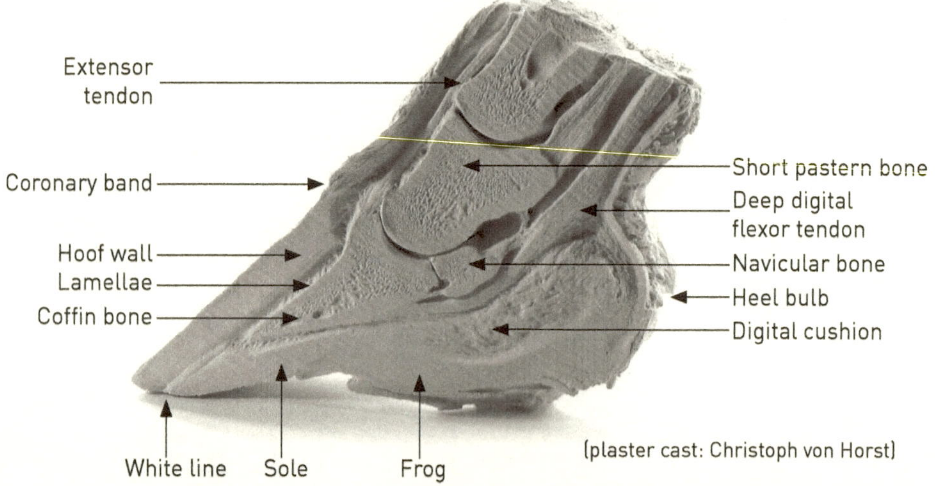

(plaster cast: Christoph von Horst)

At the bottom of the hoof are the frog, the sole, the white line and the part of the hoof wall that touches the ground. The frog provides grip to the surface, contributes to shock absorption and plays an important role in the hoof mechanism (see next question). At its centre is the central groove (or central sulcus). A healthy central groove is wide and shallow. On either side the frog is bordered by the collateral grooves. The area between the frog and the hoof wall is called the sole. The horny tissue of the sole is firm and flexible. It provides protection to the coffin bone. A healthy sole is a bit concave. The hollow shape contributes to the hoof mechanism and thus to good blood flow and shock absorption. The hoof wall and the sole are connected by the white line. Despite its name, it looks yellowish. A healthy white line is about two millimetres wide.

The hoof wall is a thick horny layer that protects the vulnerable tissues inside the hoof and gives the hoof its strength. It is not intended to support the full body weight of the horse. The front part of the hoof wall is called the toe. If we compare the hoof with a clock, the toe is the part between 10 and 2 o'clock. The back part of the hoof wall is called the heel. Each hoof wall has two heels. From there, the hoof wall bends back into the hoof. These specific parts are called the bars. They run parallel to the collateral grooves. The heel bulbs are located where the heels merge into the bulb groove.

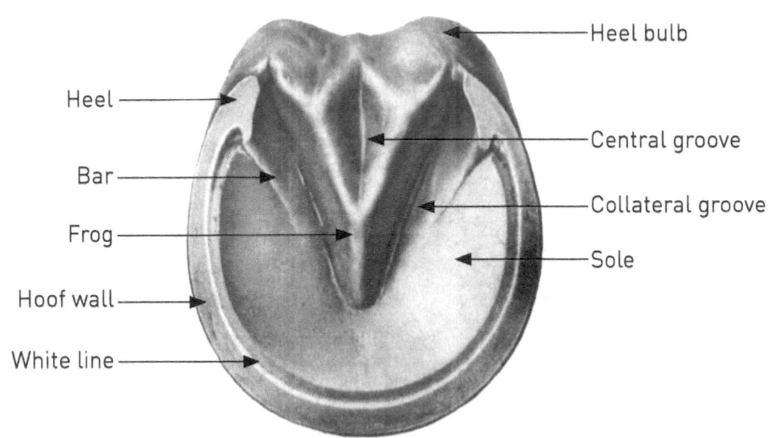

(illustration: W. Ellenberger)

THE LAMELLAR CONNECTION

The hoof wall is attached to the internal foot by a smart construction: the lamellar connection. This plays an important role in laminitis. That's why we'll take a good look at it here. The entire internal foot is covered with hoof dermis. This is a tendon-like tissue full of blood vessels and nerves. The part of the dermis that surrounds the coffin bone and the hoof cartilages is called the wall dermis. The wall dermis is covered with approximately 600 thin strips of skin tissue: the dermal lamellae. There are just as many epidermal lamellae (lamellar horn) on the inside of the hoof wall. The dermal and epidermal lamellae interlock like a kind of Velcro. In between is a wafer-thin connective tissue membrane that attaches them to each other. This membrane is called the basement membrane. It is regarded as the most important connection in the structure of the hoof. It contains proteins that ensure the connection with the horn cells of the hoof wall. These are called hemidesmosomes. The lamellar connection consists of the two types of lamella and the basement membrane together.

WHAT IS HOOF MECHANISM?

Hoof mechanism is the alternate expansion and contraction of the hoof. It makes the hoof act as a blood pump that supports the heart blood circulation. This is important for a laminitic hoof. A well-functioning blood circulation ensures the supply of oxygenated blood full of nutrients, hormones and enzymes and the removal of oxygen-depleted blood and waste products. The better the circulation in the hoof, the faster the recovery.

The hoof mechanism contributes to good shock absorption. The damaged, diseased tissues in the hoof benefit from this. Optimal hoof mechanism helps the laminitic horse to move as well as possible in its situation. Movement is important for recovery. To promote the hoof mechanism, proper, regular trimming is required. Both the use of hoof boots and housing and exercise adapted to the natural needs of the horse contribute positively.

WHAT IT IS

WHAT IS LAMINITIS?

There are many different definitions of laminitis. Clinical signs (by which you can recognise a disease) and causes are often part of these definitions. This is confusing. We should keep it as simple and as factual as possible. We'll talk about the clinical signs and causes later.

A horse has laminitis if the lamellar connection is damaged to such an extent that the dermal and the epidermal lamellae are no longer held together. The connection between the hoof wall and the coffin bone breaks down. The coffin now starts to move within the hoof capsule.

In the previous chapter, we compared the lamellar connection with Velcro. Now you know why there is a piece of detached Velcro on the cover of this book.

WHAT IS THE DIFFERENCE BETWEEN A SYMPTOM AND A CLINICAL SIGN?

A clinical sign can be determined objectively, whereas a symptom is a subjective experience by the patient. As horses cannot tell us how they experience their disease, in this book we will only use the term 'clinical sign'. Clinical signs are either measurable (e.g. fever, increased heart rate, rapid breathing) or visible (e.g. sweating, abnormal stance, stretched white line, coffin bone rotation on an X-ray).

IS LAMINITIS A HOOF DISEASE?

Even though the name would make you think differently, and even though we see the most obvious characteristics mainly in the hooves: laminitis is not a hoof disease. You could even say that laminitis itself is not an actual disease, but rather a sign that something is wrong elsewhere in the horse's body. Among others, the intestines, blood vessels and hormonal glands are often involved in the development of laminitis.

Diseases that affect multiple parts and functions of the body are called 'systemic diseases'. There is no one-to-one cause and effect. Different factors influence each other. There is often an underlying ailment, an abnormality, a deficiency or surplus, which causes the disease to strike sooner, more frequently or more severely. Laminitis is such a systemic disease.

WHAT IS SUBCLINICAL LAMINITIS?

Subclinical laminitis is a term often used incorrectly. 'Subclinical' means that there are no clinical signs to be seen or measured. Oddly enough, we come across the term with a description of easily demonstrable characteristics of laminitis, such as flares and laminitic rings (see p. 25).

True subclinical laminitis cannot be diagnosed. It is the situation in which all kind of things go wrong in the tissue cells of the lamellar connection, but this cannot yet be ascertained by a veterinarian. We also refer to this as the developmental stage. A veterinarian or hoof care provider who says that your horse has subclinical laminitis most likely means that the laminitis is in its early stages and that you need to intervene quickly to prevent it from getting worse.

CAN MY HORSE GET LAMINITIS EVEN IN WINTER?

Yes, your horse can get laminitis the whole year round. There are causes that do not care what season it is. For example, your horse can develop an infection or inflammation that leads to toxins in its body; toxins that may cause laminitis. Another example. The hay you give in winter may have been cut on a summer's day when the grass was full of sugar. If your horse is insulin resistant (see p. 36) and his blood sugar levels remain constantly too high, he may become laminitic due to the abundance of sugars in the hay.

So even though spring and autumn are more dangerous than the other two seasons, even in winter your horse can encounter an episode of laminitis. By the way, we should not confuse laminitis in winter with what we call 'winter laminitis'. On page 47 you will read what that is.

DO WILD HORSES GET LAMINITIS?

Wild horses do get laminitis, but this is less common than with domesticated horses. The living conditions of wild horses with regard to nutrition, movement environment, social interaction and natural selection are so much better than those of our domestic horses, that it is not surprising that laminitis is a typical lifestyle disease.

DOES LAMINITIS ONLY OCCUR IN HORSES?

Horses belong to the family of Equidae together with ponies, donkeys, mules and hinnies. They can all get laminitis. But other mammals such as cows, sheep, goats and pigs are not spared either. In zoos, it is deer, llamas, zebras, giraffes and even elephants and rhinos that are affected. To put it simply: if you have hooves, you can get laminitis.

HOW DOES THE LAMINITIS PROGRESS?

In the case of laminitis, the connection between the hoof wall and the coffin bone is damaged. This damage does not occur suddenly. It is a process that passes through several phases:
- The developmental phase
- The acute phase
- The chronic phase

THE DEVELOPMENTAL PHASE

This phase starts as soon as the horse is confronted with one of the possible causes and changes occur in the hoof at cellular level. Usually horses have problems with one of the systems or organs in the body before that: for example, the digestive or hormonal system. Also, sudden problems can cause the horse to become laminitic. A classic example is the horse that manages to break into the storage and open the feed bins.

The developmental phase can take between 12 and 48 hours. The lamellae start to detach during this period. The difficulty is that by definition horses show no clinical signs of laminitis in this phase so it remains unnoticed. As soon as the first signs of the disease appear, the next phase has already begun.

THE ACUTE PHASE

This phase may appear as early as after 12 hours and starts with the first clinical signs becoming visible or measurable. Almost always they are first noticeable in the front hoofs. The primary cause or causes have been present for some time and are now much more difficult to control. In fact, we are too late if we only start treating them now. This shows how very important it is to prevent laminitis. Unfortunately, the first time you have to deal with it as a horse owner, the disease usually appears completely unexpected.

The acute phase can last between 24 and 72 hours. It ends abruptly when the connection of the lamellae breaks and the coffin bone starts to let go of the hoof wall. The chronic phase has now begun.

THE CHRONIC PHASE

Once the connection between hoof wall and coffin bone fails and the lamellae let go, the horse enters the chronic phase of the disease. This phase is also called founder. The clinical signs occurring in the hooves can be easily noticed with the naked eye. The horse has to deal with constant pain and lameness. This pain and lameness vary from mild to excruciating. Later in the chronic phase, the structure and shape of the coffin bone change.

In extreme cases, the bone penetrates the sole. This is called a sole perforation (see p. 28). The horse may even lose the entire hoof capsule. This is called hoof sloughing (see p. 29). Happily enough, this does not happen very often.

The primary causes in this phase are also often chronic. Years of overweight (obesity), PPID (see p. 34) or chronic inflammation somewhere in the body are examples of this.

THERE APPEAR TO BE THREE TYPES OF LAMINITIS. WHAT ABOUT THAT?

Laminitis is an umbrella term that indicates that the connection between the hoof wall and the coffin bone is compromised. There are a bunch of possible causes for this problem. We can divide these causes into three groups, which gives us three types of laminitis:
- Hormone-related laminitis
- SIRS-related laminitis
- Traumatic laminitis

These three types of laminitis are often grouped together. This increases the risk of misdiagnosis, wrong treatment and wrong expectations. On social media, we find posts describing a specific type of laminitis followed by well-intentioned advice that is not relevant to that type. This can be detrimental if the horse owner follows the advice unthinkingly. It is therefore good to know the differences.

HORMONE-RELATED LAMINITIS

This form can be thought of as 'fat horse laminitis'. It is the most common form of laminitis. Four out of five cases (80%) fall into this category. As the name suggests, hormone-related laminitis is caused by hormonal problems. The main hormonal problems are:
- Insulin resistance/EMS
- PPID
- Corticosteroids

From page 33 we will discuss these hormonal problems.

SIRS-RELATED LAMINITIS

This form can be thought of as 'sick horse laminitis'. SIRS stands for Systemic Inflammatory Response Syndrome. This means that there is an inflammatory response of the whole body, which leads to toxins in the blood. These toxins in turn then cause the laminitis. They can be the result of inflammations and infections and of digestive problems, they can be endogenous or they can enter the body from outside. We look more closely at toxins on page 34.

TRAUMATIC LAMINITIS

This form can be thought of as 'lame horse laminitis'. The cause is a lack of oxygen in the hoof tissue. This lack of oxygen is the result of heavy, prolonged or incorrect loading of the hoofs. On page 36 we will have a look at where this overloading can originate from. Traumatic laminitis is also known as supporting limb laminitis, mechanical laminitis or road founder.

HOW DO I TELL WHICH ONE OF THE THREE IT IS?

In all three types of laminitis we see the same clinical signs, such as an increased hoof temperature, reluctance to move, leaning backwards and listless behaviour. How do you know which form of laminitis your horse has to deal with? First, you have to look at what has preceded the laminitis. If your horse broke open the feed bin and then stuffed himself with those yummy pellets full of sugar, then you can be sure that it suffers from SIRS-related laminitis. This is also the case if you know that your horse has an infectious disease (e.g. influenza) or an inflammation (e.g. eye inflammation).

If, in a manner of speaking, your horse already gets laminitis from the smell of grass alone, you should definitely be thinking in the direction of hormone-related laminitis. Your horse has an abnormal reaction to sugars. We often see signs of insulin resistance in these horses, such as a cresty neck. They usually have a high Body Condition Score as well (see the question 'What are the BCS and CNS?' on page 52). PPID (often wrongly called 'Cushing's disease') is also a notorious cause of hormone-related laminitis. Horses with PPID are generally somewhat older and can be recognised by changes in hair coat (including an abnormally thick and curly coat) and weight loss.

If you cannot identify any connection with food, it may be that there is over-straining and thus traumatic laminitis. This could be the result of stabling, overweight or efforts from the horse to avoid pain after an operation, to name but a few. Horses that are used intensively in the disciplines of endurance, reining and show jumping are at greater risk too. Incorrect trimming and shoeing may also cause traumatic laminitis.

An important and clearly observable difference is that with SIRS-related laminitis the horse looks ill, has a fever and watery diarrhea. Toxins circulate in the blood and his whole body suffers from it. This is not the case with the other two types of laminitis. Also, your vet will be able to distinguish between the different forms based on the results of a blood test. To confirm hormone-related laminitis, they will search for abnormal levels of certain hormones, such as insulin, cortisol and ACTH (see p. 34). In SIRS-related laminitis, they will find many white blood cells and antibodies in the blood.

HOW DOES THE LAMELLAR CONNECTION GET DAMAGED?

The lamellar connection can be damaged in various ways, depending on the cause and therefore the type of laminitis involved. It is beyond the scope of this book to discuss this in detail. In general, we can say that these are the two main causes of damage to the lamellar connection:
- The degradation of proteins in the basement membrane, called hemidesmosomes, which are responsible for the connection with the horny cells of the hoof wall.
- Reduced blood flow to the dermal lamellae as a result of the constriction, damage or blockage of capillaries which causes this tissue to die off.

In the book 'Laminitis : understanding, cure, prevention' you can read extensively about this subject.

WHY IS IT ALMOST ALWAYS ONLY THE FRONT HOOVES THAT GET AFFECTED?

Many clinical signs will only be seen in the front hooves. This does not mean that the hind hooves are not affected. The horse carries about 65% of its weight on its forehand, which makes the pain more pronounced there. It is also possible that the hind hooves have indeed not been damaged, while the causes of tissue damage did occur there. The horse's hindquarters are used to put the horse's strength into action. Particularly at gallop, this ensures a much better functioning hoof mechanism and thus a better blood circulation. As a result, the laminitis of the hind hooves does not develop.

Let us also not forget that there are many horses that only get shod on their front hooves. Horseshoes obstruct a good blood circulation and overload the lamellar connection. Shoes can contribute to the development of traumatic laminitis.

CAN A HORSE HAVE LAMINITIS IN JUST THE HIND HOOVES?

It does not happen very often, but it is possible. In that case, it is almost always traumatic laminitis. The horse has a chronic pain in the front of his body which causes him to overburden his hindquarters, leading to traumatic laminitis.

AND IN ONE HOOF ONLY?

That too is possible. The horse will have overloaded one leg for a long time in order to spare another part of the body. This can be seen, for example, in the case of nerve damage, a bone fracture or a joint infection. In some cases, the overburdened hoof, which is now suffers from traumatic laminitis, can cause so much trouble that the horse starts to strain the other leg again to spare the laminitic hoof. As a result, you may mistakenly think that the leg where the original problem is present is doing better.

MY HOOF CARE PROVIDER WAS TALKING ABOUT A STRETCHED WHITE LINE. WHAT IS THAT?

If the white line is wider than three millimetres, we say it is stretched. This is a characteristic of disintegration of the lamellar connection. A stretched white line is one of the first clearly visible signs that something is wrong in the hoof. Your hoof care provider will immediately come into action. They will make sure that no force exerts on the white line and the lamellar connection. They will also explain to you what you need to do to ensure that the quality of the white line and the lamellar connection improves.

WHAT IS A LAMELLAR WEDGE?

When in the chronic phase the coffin bone comes loose and starts to rotate in the hoof capsule, a space is left between the coffin bone and the hoof wall in the toe of the hoof. This space fills up with proliferating horny cells, old inflammatory blood, blood serum, necrotic (dead) hoof tissue and new inflammations. We call this whole the lamellar wedge.

WHAT IS A LAMINITIC RING?

The rotating coffin bone pulls down the tissue from which the hoof wall grows. This will create a deep ring in the hoof wall. This can already be seen a few days after the onset of laminitis. It then grows downwards from the coronary band. Based on the location of the ring in the hoof wall, we can quite accurately estimate how long ago the laminitis was acute. The re-growth of a whole new hoof wall takes about a year. So, a laminitic ring halfway down the hoof wall indicates that the laminitis struck about half a year ago.

WHAT IS A FLARE?

Flares are fanning out deformations of the hoof wall. They occur because the lamellar connection is not sufficiently capable of absorbing the mechanical forces acting on the hoof wall for a long time. Just like a stretched white line, a flare is a crystal-clear warning that the hoof is not in good health.

WHAT ARE 'ALADDIN-SLIPPERS'?

If the hoof is not properly trimmed in time and the pressure on the weakened lamellar connection is applied every time the hoof breaks over, 'Aladdin-slippers' will form. The toe of the hoof curls up. When it comes to this stage, passers-by will hopefully react and call the animal protection authorities.

WHAT ARE COFFIN BONE AND HOOF CAPSULE ROTATION?

In the chronic phase of laminitis, the angle between the coffin bone and the hoof capsule changes. Initially the bone will tilt relative to the hoof wall. In that case, the damage to the lamellar connection is limited to front of the hoof only. The bone turns, as it were, around the still-intact rear part of the lamellar connection. This happens mainly due to the force resulting from the downward pressure of the horse's weight and, to a lesser extent, the pulling force of the deep digital flexor tendon during break over of the hoof. This phenomenon is called coffin bone rotation.

At a later stage, when the lamellar connection gets damaged all around, the hoof wall will be pushed away from the coffin bone. The angle between the bone and the hoof capsule will increase further. This is called hoof capsule rotation. It happens as a result of an incorrect distribution of forces. Too long toes, a hoof wall that is too long and heels that are too high all contribute to this. The formation of the lamellar wedge also adds to this by pressing the hoof wall away from the coffin bone. For the sake of legibility, we will refer to both defects as coffin bone rotation from here on.

THE X-RAYS SHOW TEN DEGREES OF COFFIN BONE ROTATION. DOES THIS SPELL THE END OF MY HORSE?

Veterinarians generally use the following rule: a rotation of less than 5.5 degrees gives good hope; more than 11.5 degrees is a bad sign. Fortunately, there are many exceptions to these rules and they depend on the chosen treatment. A horse with a five degree coffin bone rotation, treated with therapeutic shoeing and heavy painkillers, without adaptations in movement, nutrition and housing, usually has a worse prospect than a horse with twice the amount of rotation that is properly trimmed, is given hoof boots and for which the adaptations in his living conditions do get made. The healthy growing hoof wall will be able to bring the coffin bone back to its old, normal position, no matter how big the rotation is. Of course, only under the right conditions and treatment.

Research from 2010 has shown that the speed at which the rotation increases or decreases has a much greater predictive value than the absolute degree of rotation.

THE SOLE IS FULL OF BRUISES. WHY IS THAT?

The rotating coffin bone presses on the sole from the inside. This causes bruising of the solar dermis. It shows as a moon shaped edge of red or purple sole bruises. In the case of traumatic laminitis, sole bruising occurs at an earlier stage. It is the overload that causes bruising.

Sole bruises can lead to abscesses because they reduce the quality of the sole horn. The sole becomes a little porous. Bacteria can penetrate it and cause an abscess.

WHAT IS SOLE PERFORATION?

The coffin bone can rotate, sink and press on the sole from the inside to such an extent that the sole is no longer able to withstand this pressure. The tip of the bone penetrates the sole and is visible from the outside. Sole perforation is a painful complication. Even though it looks impressive, with the proper care it can still come right. Your hoof care provider will try to optimise the position of the coffin bone as quickly as possible to prevent it from getting worse. The wound needs to be thoroughly cleaned as the risk of infection is high. The hoof is then bandaged. Hoof boots with insoles can also be useful. Where the exposed bone touches the boot, part of the insole can be cut out. The boots must always be kept clean and disinfected. The horse is given antibiotic medication. The veterinarian will regularly visit the horse to see how it is doing.

WHAT IS A SINKER?

If the lamellar connection all around the hoof is severely damaged and falls away, the coffin bone will descend vertically into the hoof capsule. This is called a sinker. The coronary band lays down flat and feels empty. In some cases, a dent in the middle of the coronary band is visible. The sole often is remarkably flat or even bulged. Sole bruising can occur.

A sinker is obviously not a good sign. Nevertheless, this can heal, provided that the correct hoof care is given, the living conditions (nutrition, housing and exercise) are improved and the cause of laminitis is found and, if possible, fixed. The growing of a healthy, connected hoof wall will bring the coffin bone back into the previous, normal position.

WHAT IS HOOF SLOUGHING?

Hoof sloughing is the loss of the hoof capsule caused by the failure of the entire connection between dermis and epidermis of the hoof. Not only the hoof wall, but also the sole, frog and hoof balls are now letting go. There have been cases of sloughing where horses have literally and figuratively got back on their feet through intensive care. However, the road to recovery is long, painful and stressful. One might seriously question whether this is still ethically justified. If your horse gets to this point and you want to take a chance, look for a very competent veterinarian and hoof care provider who both have experience with hoof sloughing. The treatment will most definitely take place in the veterinary clinic.

WHAT IS A SKI-TIP?

Bone tissue is dynamic and will adapt under pressure. The tip of the coffin bone can deform this way. This deformation, which is clearly visible on X-rays, is called a ski-tip. It can also disappear after the hoof has healed. The pressure under which it developed will then have disappeared. The new growth of a straight hoof wall will exert the necessary even pressure to force the bone back into the right shape. This process takes quite some time, about as much time as it took for the ski-tip to form in the first place. Of course, all the conditions will have to be optimal for this to happen.

CAUSES

WHAT ARE PRIMARY AND FACILITATIVE CAUSES?

Hardly ever is there a single cause for laminitis. There is, however, often a principal guilty party to blame. We call this the primary cause. It disturbs the balance in the horse's body to such an extent that the chance of complete recovery remains small as long as it is not vigorously combated. Sometimes causes accumulate without the horse becoming ill. Adding a new cause can turn the balance to the wrong side. This cause will facilitate laminitis. Hence its name, facilitative cause.

For example, a horse with chronic liver disease, such as hepatitis, will react worse to the ingestion of toxins than a horse with a healthy liver. If you are not aware of the existence of the hepatitis, you may think that a toxin has caused the laminitis. The worm treatment is blamed, while this is only a facilitative cause. This complicates treatment because the owner and care providers focus on the wrong cause.

WHAT ARE THE CAUSES OF LAMINITIS?

You know that laminitis is not a disease in itself, but rather a complex clinical phenomenon of a problem somewhere else in the body (see the question 'Is laminitis a hoof disease?' on page 17). As a result, many different causes are possible. The most common causes are problems with hormones, with the digestive system or with the blood circulation. Toxins, stress, fatty blood (hyperlipidaemia) and overburdening can also cause laminitis. We will briefly look at these causes and how they directly or indirectly can damage the lamellar connection. To be sure, please read the answer to the question 'How does the lamellar connection get damaged?' on page 23 again.
Do you want to know everything down to the last detail? The book 'Laminitis : understanding, cure, prevention' extensively describes all possible causes.

DIGESTIVE PROBLEMS

The large intestine (or colon) plays a key role in digestion. Both a good balance of gut bacteria and a healthy intestinal wall are necessary for a good functioning of the digestive system. An excessive supply of carbo-hydrates (sugars, starch and fructan) causes acidification in the colon. This leads to certain gut bacteria dying. The dying bacteria release toxins. Because the intestinal wall gets damaged by the acidification, the toxins can pass through. They go into the bloodstream where they cause blood clots (thromboses). The clots then get stuck in the smallest capillaries of the hoof dermis. The dermis now receives too little blood and partially dies. This can cause laminitis.

Another type of gut bacterium will start to proliferate. They release toxins that play a role in the breakdown of proteins in the basement membrane; proteins that are responsible for the connection with the horny cells of the hoof wall. This can also cause laminitis.

CIRCULATORY PROBLEMS

The dermal lamellae must be well supplied with blood. Proper perfusion ensures the supply of oxygenated blood, nutrients, hormones and enzymes and the removal of oxygen-depleted blood and waste products. Problems with blood circulation disrupt this process, causing the dermal lamellae to die. This damages the connection between the hoof wall and the internal foot. In other words: laminitis.

Circulatory problems are caused, among other factors, by:
- A swelling, e.g. due to an inflammation, which pinches off the blood supply
- Blood clots due to digestive problems or sudden diet changes
- Damaged capillaries in the hoof due to overloading
- Blood pressure too low, e.g. due to anaesthesia
- Some drugs, including corticosteroids

HORMONAL PROBLEMS

The most significant hormonal problems associated with laminitis are Equine Metabolic Syndrome, PPID and the use of corticosteroids.

EQUINE METABOLIC SYNDROME

In Equine Metabolic Syndrome (EMS) there is too much sugar and too much of the hormone insulin in the blood for a long time. Because the body does not respond well to the presence of insulin, these horses become insulin resistant. The large amount of blood sugar is a possible cause of laminitis. This is how it works:

1. The horse eats rapidly digestible sugars and starch.
2. The amount of sugar in the blood increases.
3. The pancreas releases insulin into the blood.
4. The cell walls of muscle cells in particular contain so-called insulin receptors.
5. Insulin 'tells' the cells via these receptors to absorb and burn the sugar.
6. If there is too much sugar in the blood too often, this is also the case for insulin.
7. If there is too much insulin in the blood too often, the receptors become 'deaf' (resistant) to the insulin.
8. Too much sugar now remains in the blood (hyperglycaemia).
9. The horse doesn't have access to that sugar, gets hungry and starts to eat more. This only makes the problem worse, because more and more sugar and insulin end up in the blood.

Hyperglycaemia causes laminitis in two ways. Firstly, it causes the breakdown of the hemidesmosomes; secondly, it causes the capillaries in the dermis to become damaged, to contract and clog.

Horses with EMS are often overweight, have a strange fat distribution (fat deposits), abnormal amounts of fat in the blood, high blood pressure and they drink and urinate more than other horses.

PPID

This abbreviation stands for Pituitary Pars Intermedia Dysfunction.
It is the condition that many people mistakenly call Cushing's disease
or syndrome. In PPID there is something wrong with a hormone gland
at the bottom of the brain: the pituitary gland. It releases too much of
certain hormones. How exactly this leads to laminitis is not yet fully
known. The main suspects are the hormones ACTH and CLIP, which
in turn cause an overproduction of the hormones cortisol and insulin. You already know the role of insulin. Cortisol causes an increase
in blood sugar levels. You've just read what too much sugar in the
blood does. Cortisol is further associated with the development and
worsening of insulin resistance and with the breakdown of cells in
the basement membrane.

CORTICOSTEROIDS

These are man-made, chemical versions of cortisol. The vet can prescribe corticosteroids against infections and inflammations. Apart from
raising blood sugar levels, corticosteroids reduce sensitivity to insulin,
just like the body's own cortisol does. In addition, they directly contribute
to the breakdown of hemidesmosomes in the basement membrane.
Corticosteroids are a good example of a facilitative cause. They will not
cause laminitis from out of nowhere. However, they can give a horse that
balances on the rim of insulin resistance the final push. There are examples of horses with respiratory tract problems (e.g. COPD) that became
laminitic after long-term use of an inhaler with beclomethasone.

Laminitis caused by equine metabolic syndrome, PPID, or the use of corticosteroids falls under hormone-related laminitis.

TOXINS

Toxins activate platelets that form clots in the blood vessels, causing them
to become clogged. In addition, they release the hormone serotonin, which
has a vasoconstrictive (narrowing) effect on the blood vessels. Both clotting and vasoconstriction restrict the blood flow to the hoof dermis and
are therefore a recipe for laminitis. On top of that, some toxins can cause

damage to the kidneys, liver or intestinal wall. Reduced functioning of the kidneys means that toxins remain in the body longer. The liver must be in good condition to eliminate excess sugar in the blood. A damaged intestinal wall allows the toxins to pass through more easily.

Other toxins can end up in the blood in all sorts of ways. Infections and inflammations are notorious sources of bacterial toxins. Keep a close eye on horses with influenza, pneumonia, eye inflammation (uveitis), udder inflammation (mastitis) or any other kind of inflammation, so that they do not also develop laminitis. The same applies to mares with a bacterial infection after placenta retention. Colic and intestinal torsion after surgery can also cause an inflammatory reaction that increases the amount of toxins in the bloodstream. In addition to these bacterial toxins, there are also fungi in hay and silage, poisonous plants, polluted drinking water, pesticides and fertilizers.

Laminitis caused by toxins falls under SIRS-related laminitis.

STRESS
Prolonged and increased stress causes hormonal, blood sugar level and circulatory problems. It disturbs production of cortisol. In stressful situations, this hormone converts proteins and fat into sugar. This causes blood sugar levels to rise. This also happens because more of the stress hormone adrenaline is produced. Adrenaline reduces the sensitivity to insulin, so that more sugar remains in the blood. Adrenaline also has a constrictive effect on the blood vessels. So do the stress hormones norepinephrine and dopamine.

FATTY BLOOD
The popular name of hyperlipidaemia indicates that there is now too much fat in the blood. This can lead to vasoconstriction in the hooves. It gets almost tedious to keep repeating it, but the reduced blood flow causes the dying off of hoof tissue (the hoof dermis, dermal lamellae and the basement membrane). Laminitis can strike or the condition can worsen. When a horse suddenly has nothing or much less to eat this problem can also occur. For example, when sudden heavy snowfall makes grazing impossible. In late

pregnant or lactating mares blood fattening can also occur, especially if they don't get enough food to compensate for the pregnancy or milk yield. Ponies, donkeys and miniature horses, ponies that are too fat and horses with PPID are at risk too.

MECHANICAL OVERLOAD (TRAUMA)

Besides hormone-related and SIRS-related laminitis, there is also traumatic laminitis (see p. 22). The cause is heavy, prolonged, repetitive strain on the hooves, often on a hard surface. Overloading of the hooves can be caused by, among other things:

- Incorrect trimming (underrun heels, bars or toe too long)
- Toe first landing (e.g. due to pain somewhere else in the hoof or body, like navicular syndrome, a hoof abscess or back pain)
- Shoeing
- Working for a prolonged period of time on a hard surface (carriage horses, police horses)
- Overweight
- Stabling
- Long distance transport
- The horse trying to avoid pain (e.g. after an operation)

The hoof tissue is simply not able to withstand overloading. The capillaries in the hoof get damaged or pinched. This leads to insufficient blood flow and thereby oxygen shortage in the hoof dermis and dermal lamellae. Result: mechanical laminitis, as we sometimes call traumatic laminitis.

WHAT IS INSULIN RESISTANCE?

Insulin is the hormone that ensures that body cells absorb sugar from the blood. In case of insulin resistance, the cells do not respond well to insulin. Sugar is not absorbed well and the blood sugar level remains too high (hyperglycaemia). Insulin resistance is an important clinical sign of Equine Metabolic Syndrome (EMS).

WHAT IS EMS?

EMS is the abbreviation for Equine Metabolic Syndrome. It is the equine variety of type 2 diabetes in humans. On page 33 is explained what it means.

WHAT IS THE DIFFERENCE BETWEEN INSULIN RESISTANCE AND EMS?

EMS is effectively a collection of disorders. These are mainly insulin resistance, weight problems, high blood pressure and deviating blood fat levels. Since insulin resistance is the most important characteristic of EMS, we also call it insulin resistance syndrome. Obesity and insulin resistance influence each other mutually. Obesity causes insulin resistance; insulin resistance causes obesity. So, there is a difference between EMS and insulin resistance, but this is mainly theoretical.

MY VET MENTIONED OBESITY AND ADIPOSITY. WHAT ARE THEY AND WHAT IS THE DIFFERENCE?

There are two types of fat horses: fat due to overeating and fat due to hormonal problems. The first type has a big belly and is heavier than it should be. This horse is obese. Dietary changes and exercise work wonders. The second type has a strange body fat distribution. There are fat deposits above the eyes, on the neck, shoulders, on top of the rump, above the tail and around the sheath or udder. This form of overweight is called adiposity. Adiposity is often found in horses with EMS. Of course, a horse can have both obesity and adiposity.

THERE'S NOT JUST ONE KIND OF SUGAR, IS THERE?

We're talking about sugar in the horse's diet, but we actually should use the broader term carbohydrates. This is because there are carbohydrates that are not sugar, such as fructan, starch and dietary fibre. Because you will often come across the different kinds of carbohydrates in this book and beyond, we will briefly discuss them here.

These types of carbohydrates can be distinguished:
- Simple and dual carbohydrates, such as glucose (dextrose), fructose (fruit sugar) and sucrose (beet sugar). These are also known as fast carbohydrates.
- Fructan. There are different kinds of fructans, but in this book we collectively call them 'fructan' for convenience.
- Complex carbohydrates, such as starch and dietary fibre (a.o. cellulose).

In your forage analysis results, on labels of horse feed and in the rest of this book, you will also find these abbreviations of the different types of carbohydrates:
- ESC: Ethanol-Soluble Carbohydrates = simple and double sugars
- WSC: Water-Soluble Carbohydrates = ESC and fructan
- NSC: Non-Structural Carbohydrates = WSC and starch
- SC: Structural Carbohydrates = dietary fibre

WHAT IS FRUCTAN?

If more sugar is available than needed for growth, the grasses that grow in our fields store it as fructan, to be used in better times in terms of growing conditions. This is the case, for example, during a cool night when growth comes to a complete standstill. Storage also occurs when other growth factors, such as enough water, the right temperature and nutrients, are not sufficiently present.

In addition, fructan serves as a kind of antifreeze. When the temperature drops below minus ten (14 °F), fructan is converted back into sugar. Just as sugar water freezes less easily than pure water, the plant will also be better protected against frost. You will read about the link between fructan and laminitis in the following answer.

DON'T HORSES OFTEN GET LAMINITIS FROM FRUCTAN?

No, although that was thought for a long time. It is true that the consumption of large amounts of fructan could have an effect on the development or worsening of laminitis, but only in the case of SIRS-related laminitis. This type of laminitis occurs in only about 10% of all cases and even then, it can be caused by all kinds of other things.

Let's then look at what role fructan does play. Fructan is a WSC made up of long chains of mainly fructose molecules. Horses do not have the right enzymes in their digestive tract to digest fructan. The bacteria in the colon do this for them by fermentation. Volatile fatty acids are released in the process. For horses that are only fed roughage, these fatty acids are the main source of energy. Too much fructan in the large intestine causes the production of fatty acids that is higher than the blood can take up. This causes acidification in the intestine. Now what happens is described on page 32 under 'Digestive problems'. Let's briefly repeat: intestinal wall damage in combination with dying bacteria that release toxins and proliferating bacteria that cause important proteins in the basement membrane to break down.

WHAT IS STRESSED GRASS?

If all conditions are right for the plant (sunny, temperature above five degrees Celsius, enough water and nutrients), sugars and fructan (WSC) are used for growth. If one or more of these factors are lacking, the grass will make and store more WSC. We call grass 'stressed' at this stage. A combination of sunny weather during the day and low night temperatures is the perfect recipe for stressed grass. Lots of sunlight combined with too low a daytime temperature or too few nutrients also scores high.

I THOUGHT ONLY SPRING WAS DANGEROUS. NOW IT IS AUTUMN AND MY HORSE IS SUDDENLY LAMINITIC. HOW IS THAT POSSIBLE?

In autumn, when the night frost returns and the sun shines brightly during the day, the risk of stressed grass is greater. Depending on how much grass there is left in the pasture, some people already start feeding hay. This hay may have been harvested at a time when the grass was full of sugars. Those sugars are now in the hay.

In addition, the way in which we exercise our horses often changes abruptly in autumn. The summer holidays with lots of time to go out for long rides are over. Many horses suddenly come to a standstill. With less exercise in combination with feed full of carbohydrates, laminitis is immediately lurking.

Horses with PPID have a larger amount of the hormone ACTH in their blood in late summer and early autumn. This increases the production of the hormone cortisol, which in turn increases blood sugar levels. The hormone CLIP is derived from ACTH. The production of CLIP is therefore also higher during this period. There are indications that CLIP is responsible for the production of insulin by the pancreas.

THE GRASS IS VERY SHORT. YET MY HORSE GOT LAMINITIS. HOW IS THAT EVEN POSSIBLE?

If the flowering of the grass plant is disturbed by, for example, sudden frost, hail, voracious insects or cattle trampling the grass, the grass seed does not develop. The carbohydrates normally used to develop seed then remain in the stems. This also applies to grass that has been nibbled off to the ground.

It thus contains a lot of carbohydrates. Your horse doesn't know this and will continue grazing until he is no longer hungry. If he does so with this short, sugary grass, he runs a greater risk of developing laminitis. So, turning a laminitic horse out on short grass as a dietary measure, without adding low-energy hay, is not a good idea.

IS PPID THE SAME AS CUSHING'S DISEASE?

The terms PPID and Cushing's disease are often confused or used as synonyms. On page 34 you have read what PPID is. With Cushing's disease there is also something wrong with the pituitary gland. However, the problem then lies in just another part of the pituitary gland. As a result, the disease progresses in a different way than in PPID. It looks a lot like PPID, but it is not the same. In contrast to dogs and humans, Cushing's disease is almost non-existent in horses. Let us call a spade a spade from now on.

WHAT IS ACTH?

ACTH is a hormone secreted by the pituitary gland. In horses with PPID, too much ACTH is present in the blood. Incidentally, this is also the case in horses that are in pain or under stress. From the end of July to the beginning of November, ACTH levels are higher in all horses, usually with a peak in September/October. We call this the seasonal rise.

WHAT IS CORTISOL?

You have seen cortisol being mentioned a couple of times now. The adrenal glands secrete this hormone to quickly convert proteins and fats into glucose in stressful situations. The muscles can make good use of this fast sugar if the horse has to run for its life when there is a hungry lion around. Things are a little less exciting for our domestic horse. The glucose increases the blood sugar level. Cortisol has a vasoconstrictive effect and is associated with the development and worsening of insulin resistance. In addition, it plays a role in the breakdown of the hemidesmosomes in the basement membrane.

DOES MY HORSE HAVE EMS OR IS IT PPID?

Adiposity (see p. 37), laminitis and insulin resistance are clinical signs of both EMS and PPID. These are the differences:

- EMS usually starts at a lower age, PPID is more - but not exclusively - of an aging disease.
- Clinical signs characteristic of PPID, such as thick and curly coats, are absent in EMS.
- In horses with PPID, it has been shown that there is too much ACTH in the blood when not in pain or under stress and not during the seasonal rise.

Obviously, horses can also have both conditions.

MY HORSE IS GIVEN CORTICOSTEROIDS. COULD THIS LEAD TO LAMINITIS?

It is possible, but it does not happen very often. Usually there is something the matter with your horse. Go back to page 34, where this is explained.

CAN TOO MUCH PROTEIN IN THE GRASS PROVOKE A BOUT OF LAMINITIS?

For a long time, it was thought that the proteins were the big evildoers when overeating. We now know that this is not true. Excess protein is broken down and drained away through the urine. It is true, however, that ammonia is released during this breakdown. This puts too much strain on the liver and kidneys. The ammonia also disturbs the bacterial culture in the large intestine. So, it can play a small role, but it will certainly not be the main cause.

MY MARE WILL SOON HAVE A FOAL.
WHAT'S THE STORY WITH THE PLACENTA AND LAMINITIS?

If the placenta is not completely expulsed within two hours after birth, a bacterial infection can occur. This can cause SIRS-related laminitis. This is one of the reasons why laminitis is relatively common in broodmares.

MY HORSE HAS SURVIVED A SEVERE COLIC ATTACK AND NOW IT HAS
LAMINITIS. IS THERE A LINK?

When the intestine is twisted due to colic, the blood supply to the intestinal wall will be pinched off. The intestinal wall becomes damaged and toxins will pass through more easily. The amount of toxins is already higher because colic causes an inflammatory reaction in which these are released. This can lead to SIRS-related laminitis. If the intestinal wall was already damaged by acidification (see the question 'Digestive problems' on page 32), the problems accumulate and the risk of laminitis only increases.

MY HORSE GOT LAMINITIS AFTER DRINKING A LOT OF WATER.
HOW IS THAT POSSIBLE?

Drinking too much water all at once affects the intestinal flora. Many bacteria die off in the large intestine. As a result of the death of these bacteria, toxins are released that leave the intestine and end up in the bloodstream. There they cause small clots that eventually get stuck in the capillaries of the hoof dermis. These microvessels now get too little blood and partially die off. This can cause laminitis. It is often said that too cold water can also have this effect, but this is simply not true.

COULD A VACCINE OR A WORM TREATMENT BE THE CAUSE?

Vaccinations and worm cures could be seen as toxins and thus contribute to the development of SIRS-related laminitis. In practice, this hardly ever occurs as a facilitative cause. If you suspect that there are already quite a few toxins in your horse's body, you would do well to wait a while before vaccinating and deworming. Toxins should not be piling up.

IS MY HORSE AT GREATER RISK?

If your horse is in one of these categories, it will be at greater risk of getting laminitis:
- Pony breeds originating from arid or cold areas and donkeys, as they have a tendency to develop obesity and insulin resistance.
- Overweight horses
- Horses with insulin resistance, EMS or PPID
- Older horses, as they might have been exposed to risk factors longer than younger horses and often have had laminitis before. PPID is also more common in older horses.
- Warmblood and thoroughbred horses. These breeds often have thin and flat soles, which increases the risk of traumatic laminitis.
- Large draught horses
- Horses suffering from another disease, an acute infection or chronic inflammation somewhere else in the body
- Mares that recently had a foal
- All horses whose natural needs are insufficiently met, in terms of housing, movement, nutrition and hoof care. And unfortunately, there are still very many.

OKAY, SO STRESS IS BAD FOR MY LAMINITIC HORSE. BUT HOW DO I PREVENT STRESS?

On page 35 you have learned why stress is not good for your horse. There is a laundry list of stress factors that you could reduce or eliminate:

- Pain
- Transportation
- Competition
- Chronic worm infestation
- Veterinarian consultation, rushed or grumpy farrier, dentist
- Poorly fitting saddle
- Weaning too young
- Starting young horses too young
- Monotonous training
- Lack of social interaction: no herd or alone in box
- Restless living environment. For example, a busy livery yard or a pasture next to a motorway.
- Mourning. Two horses that have grown up together or that have chosen each other as buddy who are suddenly separated.
- Radiation from antennas and high voltage cables

IS MY HORSE MORE LIKELY TO GET LAMINITIS AGAIN NOW THAT HE HAS HAD IT ONCE?

Horses that have had laminitis not so long ago are indeed more likely to return to it. This may be because the damaged dermal lamellae are more sensitive to the conditions that cause laminitis. Your horse is also more likely to have painful hooves because tissues and nerves have been damaged. Pain causes blood sugar levels to rise and blood vessels to constrict. These are two risk factors. In addition, it may well be that the primary or facilitative causes have not all completely disappeared. So, keep a close eye on your horse and pay a lot of attention to the prevention of a new episode of laminitis.

ONE OF MY PONIES KEEPS GETTING LAMINITIS, THE OTHER DOESN'T. HOW IS THAT POSSIBLE?

Two ponies live in the same field, get the same food and exercise and have had the same hoof care provider for years. And yet one of them is always getting laminitis. That is very frustrating. Apparently, there is still an aspect that you, your veterinarian or your hoof care provider overlook. Start by checking whether all these factors are really the identical. Maybe this pony doesn't move as much around the field as his meadow buddy does. Don't you unknowingly have a preference for the other pony when going out for a hike? Also ask your hoof care provider if they might be trimming one differently from the other. Isn't this pony shod whilst the other one goes barefoot?

It could also be that he has an underlying problem that you haven't discovered yet. An inflammation or a chronic disease, for example. Maybe he is insulin resistant or has PPID without you knowing it. It is also possible that a number of facilitative causes have piled up and that the pile is now falling over. Or perhaps you are focusing on the cause that you do know and have under control, but therefore overlook another cause. You could also ask for a second opinion from another vet.

Take a close look at the following factors too:
- Weight, BCS and CNS (see p. 52)
- Drugs, vaccinations, worm treatment, supplements
- Nutritional and housing changes, grazing times, how the pony gets its exercise

You might discover patterns that can help you find hidden causes. Don't look for more than one cause at a time. Concentrate on one thing. If that' s not it, move on to the next one.

IS LAMINITIS HEREDITARY?

Laminitis itself is not hereditary. However, EMS can be. Some breeds have a tendency to develop EMS. These include Appaloosas, Welsh, Exmoor, New Forest and Shetland ponies, cobs, Icelandic and Arabian horses. The same applies to certain bloodlines in other breeds. Hoof shape can also be partially hereditary. A less good hoof shape could contribute to the development of traumatic laminitis.

WHAT IS WINTER LAMINITIS?

Insulin resistant horses can suffer from painful hooves in winter. This is known as winter laminitis, although in fact it is not really laminitis. Something like 'winter-related hoof pain syndrome' would be a better name. Sudden, rapidly dropping temperatures in winter cause the adrenal glands to produce more cortisol. Cortisol is a hormone that has a constrictive effect on the blood vessels. The blood flow to the hooves decreases. In addition, the body produces more thyroid hormones to fight the cold, reducing blood flow even more. The poor circulation causes pain that gets worse when the horse has to walk over frozen, bumpy surfaces. Because pain and the associated stress cause an increase in cortisol production, this creates a vicious circle.

Especially horses with PPID or EMS often suffer from winter laminitis. This is because all horses with EMS are insulin resistant, which is also the case for 60% horses with PPID. Horses with damaged blood vessels, because they have been laminitic in the past, are also at greater risk.

DIAGNOSIS

DOES MY HORSE HAVE LAMINITIS?

Even though it is usually obvious that a horse has laminitis, the diagnosis has to be made by a veterinarian. This sounds self-evident, but it happens all too often that the hoof care provider, trainer or yard manager states that your horse is laminitic when it is not. If your horse actually does have laminitis, these people do not know at what stage of the disease is and how serious the situation is. For example, they cannot carry out a blood test or interpret the results of such a test properly. Neither can they take X-rays or consult a radiologist if these photos raise any questions. So, if you think that your horse has laminitis, you should call the vet. Your second call should be to the hoof care provider. They may not make the diagnosis, but they will have to come into action quickly all the same.

MY HOOF CARE PROVIDER HAS SAID THAT MY HORSE HAS LAMINITIS. DO I STILL HAVE TO CALL THE VET?

Certainly not every horse owner will do this, but it is still highly advisable. Laminitis is a medical problem. Even though your hoof care provider has seen and successfully helped numerous horses, he is not a veterinarian. However, it is very beneficial if he and the vet consult each other and work together if necessary. This will help the vet to make a better diagnosis. The hoof care provider will also be able to do his job better. X-rays, results of blood tests and a clearly established cause will be more than welcome.

HOW CAN I RECOGNIZE LAMINITIS MYSELF?

Especially in the acute phase there are signs that a horse owner can recognise. If you notice one or more of these, take immediate first aid measures (see the question 'What should I do if I think that my horse has laminitis?' on page 58) and call your vet.

Horses with acute laminitis often show one or more of these signs:

- Muscle tremors, sweating, dilated pupils, widened nostrils, ears stiffly turned backwards
- Rapid or irregular and erratic breathing (80-100 breaths per minute)
- Increased body temperature (40-41 °C/104-106 °F)
- Strong and rapid pulse (80-120 beats per minute), pulsations
- Increased hoof temperature for a longer period of time (over 30 °C/86 °F for 24 hours)
- Sometimes a slightly stretched white line can already be noticed
- Stiff or not wanting to move at all, difficulty with turns, more lame on a hard surface than on a soft one
- Laminitic stance (leaning backwards), shifting of weight, sometimes the feet are alternately lifted, lie down a lot

HOW DO I KNOW IF MY HORSE IS IN PAIN?

Pain assessment in a horse is not easy. It is like kicking down an open door, but horses cannot tell us whether and how much they experience pain. They do not necessarily want us to know either. In the wild, you will soon be a target for predators if you show that you are weak. Nevertheless, it is important that you recognise in time whether your horse is in pain. The sooner you intervene in laminitis, the greater the chance of a quick recovery.

Some of the characteristics mentioned above already show that the horse is in pain. In particular, leaning backwards in the laminitic stance helps the horse to feel less pain in its front hooves. A horse that sighs and moans or shows withdrawn behaviour is also in pain. Pay particular attention to how your horse reacts differently than usual. You know him best, so you recognise almost intuitively when something is wrong.

WHAT IS THE LAMINITIC STANCE?

With the laminitic stance the horse tries to alleviate pain in his front hooves by leaning backwards. The hoof wall puts pressure on the front of the hoof. This is painful in the case of laminitis because the dermis and its dermal lamellae are damaged. Painful pressure on the coronary band and pressure from the tip of the coffin bone on the sole also get less when the horse is in this position.

The laminitic stance not only reduces pain, but also helps to heal. It takes the pressure off the dermal lamellae, which can then recover better. The hoof mechanism improves and so does the blood circulation. Less pain means less cortisol; less cortisol ultimately results in a slightly lower blood sugar level. This is beneficial in many cases of laminitis.

WHAT ARE PULSATIONS?

Inflammation of the dermal lamella is a clinical sign of acute laminitis. When blood platelets are activated by this inflammation, they bind and clot. These small clots clog the capillaries in the hoof. The platelets also release a substance that has a constrictive effect on the blood vessels. A swelling of inflammatory fluid also partially pinches the blood vessels. These three things together hinder the blood supply to the hoof. Blood accumulates in the arteries. The heartbeat can now be felt as strong pulsations.

HOW DO I TAKE MY HORSE'S DIGITAL PULSE?

The digital pulse can be felt in the artery in the groove between the tendons at the back of the lower leg. Slightly lower, the artery continues into the fetlock. The pulse can be felt there as well, just like on the coronary band. The index finger and middle finger combined are the most sensitive. Place them flat on the artery and leave them like this for a few seconds. Count the number of pulses for 15 seconds and multiply that number by four. This way you will know the number of pulses per minute.

WHAT ARE THE BCS AND CNS?

BCS stands for 'Body Condition Score'. It is a rating system that the veterinarian can use to assess the body condition of horses. A score of one or two is for horses that are (too) skinny, three and four are reasonable and good, five and six is bad news especially for insulin-resistant horses. It means they are (way) too fat.

CNS stands for 'Cresty Neck Score'. It is a rating system used to evaluate the amount of fat on a horse's neck and thereby its obesity. The scale is six points where a score of four and higher is not good.

HOW DO I MEASURE THE NECK SIZE OF MY HORSE?

The neck size indicates whether your horse reacts well to dietary changes, more exercise or certain supplements. It is therefore useful if you can take measurements of your horse's neck size yourself. Measure with a flexible tape measure in the middle of the neck, between the crown of the head and withers. The neck should be relaxed while the head is up. Write down the results after each measurement. This way you can see if there are any changes. An increase in neck circumference is also a good predictor of the risk of a new bout of laminitis. If you see this happening, then hopefully you will be able to do something in time.

HOW DOES THE VETERINARIAN MAKE THE DIAGNOSIS?

The diagnosis will include at least two of the following elements:
- Anamnesis: mapping the history and circumstances of the disease. The vet will ask you a lot of questions.
- Clinical examination: identifying as many clinical signs as possible. These include taking temperature, measuring pulse and respiratory rate, but also using a hoof tester and gait evaluation/lameness assessment.

- Medical imaging: e.g. X-rays and thermal images.
- Differential diagnosis: method of diagnosing a disease by excluding other conditions that have similar clinical signs. Blood tests play an important part in this.

WHAT IS THE OBEL GRADING SYSTEM?

This is a system used to classify the degree of lameness. The scale runs from 0 to 4, where only Obel 0 stands for 'all movement is without problems'. The higher the score, the more lame the horse is. The veterinarian and the hoof care provider can use this system to monitor the healing progress. A horse going from Obel 4 to Obel 3 is on its way up.

The classification is as follows:
0. All movement is without problems.
1. Weight shifting from one foot to the other or incessantly lifting of the feet. At the trot a stabbing or shortened stride.
2. Stiff movement at a walk. A foot can be lifted off the ground without difficulty.
3. Horse moves reluctantly and resists attempts to lift the feet.
4. Horse refuses to move.

WHY DOES THE VETERINARIAN USE HOOF TESTERS?
CAN THE HOOF CARE PROVIDER DO THIS TOO?

Hoof testers can be used to detect sensitivity by exerting pressure on certain areas of the hoof. The veterinarian uses this tool as part of the clinical examination. It looks easy, but still requires experience in both using the tool and interpreting the horse's reaction. Hoof testers therefore belong in the hands of a vet and not in those of the hoof care provider.

DO I NEED TO HAVE X-RAYS?
WHERE CAN I HAVE THEM TAKEN AND HOW MUCH DOES IT COST?

X-rays are useful:
- To determine the severity of the laminitis and the stage of the disease. For example, coffin bone rotation or a sinker can be made clearly visible, as can a ski-tip (see p. 29).
- To see possible traces of previous laminitis.
- To assess the progress of the healing process.

The costs may vary considerably from one clinic to another. On average, an X-ray costs forty pounds. Please bear in mind that the vet sometimes wants to have several photos: from different sides, with the hoof loaded and unloaded. X-rays can be taken at the clinic or at your own location. In that case there will be additional travel costs. Ask in advance what it is going to cost, so you won't be faced with any surprises.

WHAT IS A THERMAL IMAGE?

Thermography can be used to visualise heat radiation from the body. With this technique we can map out processes such as blood flow and inflammation. Taking a good thermal image requires a lot of experience from the photographer. A little cold draught can already distort the outcome. Interpretation of the photo can also be difficult. What is found is not always important for the diagnosis. Thermography is a useful additional tool for making the diagnosis, but do not overestimate it.

WHAT BLOOD TESTS IS THE VET GOING TO CARRY OUT?

A blood test is a good starting point if obvious causes, such as the emptying of a feed bin, are ruled out. It gives clear and factual information about:

- Hormone and blood sugar levels. Insulin, glucose, cortisol and ACTH are measured to determine or exclude EMS or PPID.
- Vitamin and mineral deficiencies or surpluses. When it comes to minerals, blood tests are not always helpful; some deficiencies are not visible in the blood.
- Reduced liver or kidney function.
- Fatty blood (see p. 35).
- Dehydration.

It is a good idea to have the blood test done again after a few months. The vet will then do the same tests, under the same conditions as the first time. The results are therefore comparable and show whether there is an improvement or not.

WHAT ARE REFERENCE RANGES OR NORMAL LAB VALUES?

We use reference ranges for blood tests. These are two extremes within which the results are acceptable or normal. We therefore also call them normal lab values. The vast majority of healthy horses fall within these values. If blood tests give a result that is outside the range (both higher and lower), the vet will see reason to confirm his suspicion that he had, based on the anamnesis and clinical examination. If it stays within the normal values, he will continue his search. If all results are within the normal values, this will disprove his suspicion.

COULDN'T IT BE NOT SOMETHING ELSE?

There are hoof problems that give complaints that may be reminiscent of laminitis, especially if they occur in both front hooves at the same time:
- Navicular syndrome/caudal hoof pain syndrome
- Sole bruising, abscess
- Advanced white line disease (see p. 120)
- Keratoma (abnormal horn growth on the inside of the hoof wall)
- Coffin joint inflammation (arthritis)
- Osteoarthritis
- Cysts in the coffin bone or navicular bone
- Coffin bone fracture

Then there are diseases that show stiffness and reluctance to move, just as we know in laminitis. These are tetanus, rabies, Monday disease, pneumonia and abdominal pain (e.g. a chronically inflamed or irritated appendix).

TREATMENT

CAN A HORSE BE CURED OF LAMINITIS?

Remember when we said that laminitis itself is not really a disease, but
a sign that something is wrong somewhere else in the horse's body?
So, whether laminitis can be cured will depend on us being able to find out
what problem is causing it and whether we can solve it. Sometimes that is
easy. Your horse breaks out of the field and feasts on a pile of apples under your neighbour's apple tree. The large amount of sugars in it causes
the laminitis. From now on, simply make sure that this can't happen again.
In other cases, it is not that simple. The underlying disease can be incurable, such as PPID. You will then be faced with medication, dietary changes
and the treatment of complications, such as hoof abscesses.

You will always have to start a rehabilitation programme. The success of
this depends to a large extent on the severity of the laminitis. The skills of
your vet and your hoof care provider also play an important role. Last but
definitely not least, it comes down to you. To what extent are you prepared
to improve your horse's living conditions? Nutrition, housing and exercise
usually need to be addressed. Do you have the time, the money and the
inclination to do so?

In short, we can say that there is a good chance that laminitis cures completely if you are there on time, if the cause is found and eliminated as much
as possible, if the damage to the hooves is not too severe, if the hooves are
properly and regularly trimmed and if you work on all aspects to perfect the
living conditions of your horse.

WHAT SHOULD I DO IF I THINK THAT MY HORSE HAS LAMINITIS?

Step 1: Call the veterinarian.
Step 2 and onwards:

- Take your horse off the pasture. Put him in the paddock or riding arena.
- Make sure he can lie down comfortably.
- Cool the hooves and lower legs (see p. 60).
- Provide clean drinking water.
- Provide low-energy, coarse hay, preferably soaked in warm water (see p. 61).
- Do not give food that contains a lot of sugar or starch; not even a handful of grain or half an apple.
- Provide a salt lick or give two tablespoons of iodised salt daily.
- Give magnesium to increase insulin sensitivity (see p. 72).
  If later it turns out that your horse is not insulin resistant, then giving magnesium is not bad for your horse, unless he has kidney problems.
- Call a hoof care provider to trim the hooves and pull the shoes if your horse is shod.
- A farrier who suggests therapeutic shoes, who doesn't want to shorten the hoof wall, who wants to raise the heels or offers other old-fashioned solutions, is best kept away from your horse.
- Make emergency insoles (see p. 60) or use hoof boots.
- Ask your vet about the possibilities of pain medication.

DOES MY HORSE HAVE TO BE HOSPITALISED?

Depending on the state of your horse's health, the veterinarian may want to treat your horse in the clinic. Horses that are so heavily laminitic that they cannot stand for long or even get up at all are better off in the clinic than at home. This is especially true if there are serious complications such as sole perforation or hoof sloughing. A horse with such problems needs more care and supervision of the healing process than you can offer outside a clinic.

IS BOX REST NECESSARY?

Box rest is hardly ever a solution. In fact, it is often one of the causes. Your horse cannot move sufficiently in its box. Because of this, the hooves are not well supplied with blood. Then there is the stress with its negative effects. So put your horse in a paddock or arena during the acute phase of laminitis. In the absence of a paddock you might be able to create an acceptable temporary solution by fencing off part of the yard. If this is all impossible, you could maybe join several stables to create a bigger space.

But... don't do this if he is so bad that all movement causes pain. Ask your vet about pain medication. Discuss the possibilities of hoof boots with your hoof care provider. There are therapeutic boots that are specially made for laminitic horses. Of course, there are also situations in which box rest is more important for the recovery of the underlying problem. Consult with your veterinarian on how to reduce this period to a minimum.

MY HORSE IS LYING DOWN FOR SUCH A LONG TIME THAT HE GETS PRESSURE SORES. WHAT SHOULD I DO?

Apply a thick layer of bedding. Preferably your horse is lying on 30 centimetres (12") of straw or sawdust with a top layer of peat moss. Keep the spot where it is lying clean. Remove dirty bedding, urine and manure immediately. Shake up the bedding a few times a day. Make sure the ambient temperature is low. A recumbent horse can hardly get rid of its heat, especially if it has fever. If the horse sweats less, the risk of developing pressure sores is smaller. Every 2 to 3 hours you need to help your horse to change position. Try to keep the horse in the sternal (chest) position as much as possible. If any pressure sores do occur, clean them and apply a greasy, unscented skin ointment. When the time has come for you to provide this care, you should ask your vet if your horse is not better off in the clinic.

WHAT IS COLD THERAPY?

You can apply cold therapy as a first aid measure. It slows down the development of the disease because the metabolism in the cells of the dermal lamellae slows down. It also reduces inflammation and pain.

HOW DO I COOL THE HOOVES?

Cooling with a garden hose, cold therapy compresses (gel packs) or cooling ointment does not work well enough. Place the hooves in buckets or soaking boots with ice water. The deeper the hooves are in it, the better. Keep adding crushed ice and replacing the warmed-up water to keep the temperature low. A lower limit of 2 °C (35.5 °F) for a minimum of 24 and a maximum of 72 hours is safe. In consultation with your vet you can cool longer than 72 hours.

HOW DO I MAKE EMERGENCY INSOLES?

A gardening kneeling pad can quickly be transformed into emergency insoles to temporarily protect your horse's painful hooves:
- Make sure the hoof is clean, dry and preferably correctly trimmed.
- Place the hoof on the pad.
- Use a marker to trace the outline of the hoof on the pad.
- Cut it out.
- Lift the hoof and place the insole under it. Use duct tape to attach. First use a strip of tape going from the side of the hoof the other side, keeping the insole in place.
- Lay a gauze on the heel bulbs to protect them from the glue from the duct tape. Now wrap the hoof and insole with tape. Be careful not to tape the coronary band.

DO I NEED TO STIMULATE BLOOD CIRCULATION IN THE HOOVES?

If your horse is suddenly laminitic, blood circulation should not be stimulated. At the onset of the acute phase, if you don't yet know exactly what the cause is, it is possible that enzymes in the blood that affect the basement membrane are the culprit. A higher blood flow then results in a larger supply of these enzymes.

As soon as your vet gives the green light, stimulating the blood flow is a good idea. It ensures the supply of oxygenated blood full of nutrients and the removal of oxygen-depleted blood and waste products. This is necessary to allow the tissues in the hoof to recover well and quickly.

HOW DO I DO THIS?

Movement is still the best way to increase blood flow. Let your horse move carefully (!) as soon as the veterinarian or hoof care provider says this is possible. Preferably use hoof boots with soft insoles and make absolutely sure that your horse is properly trimmed.

The vet may prescribe vasodilator drugs (that widen the blood vessels), such as acepromazine or pentoxifylline. Some plants are said to increase blood flow. These include buckwheat, nettle, yarrow, hawthorn, cleavers and jiaogulan. There are also droplets with substances from these and other plants in them that are supposed to increase the blood flow. How well this really works is open to debate.

DO I NEED TO SOAK HAY?
HOW DO I DO THAT?

If you don't have low-energy hay (less than 10% carbohydrates), you can soak and rinse your hay. This way about half of the fast sugars and fructan (the water-soluble carbohydrates or WSC, see page 38) can be removed from the hay in about an hour. Rinsing in more or fresh water ensures even more washing out. Warm water rinses twice as fast as cold water. Unfortunately, it also removes important minerals and vitamins. Soaking between 15 and 30 minutes gives the best ratio between rinsed out WSC and preservation of minerals and vitamins. The use of a broad-spectrum supplement (balancer, see page 92) is recommended. It is practical to soak in a large tub or wheelbarrow. Do not soak more hay than the horse can eat in one day. Wet hay can easily become mouldy. Throw away the water after soaking.

DO HORSES EVEN LIKE WET HAY?

Your horse will not be mad excited in the beginning, but after a while he will eat it. Hunger is still the best sauce. In case he really doesn't like it, you could mix it with beet pulp or a bit of dry hay, which you then reduce over a couple of days.

DO I STILL HAVE TO SOAK THE HAY IN WINTER?

As long as you don't know how high the amount of carbohydrates in the hay is, it's better to be safe than sorry. The hay may have been harvested at a time when the grass was full of sugars. Sugars that are now in the hay. This is particularly likely with first cut hay.

CAN HAYLAGE OR BEET PULP ALSO BE SOAKED?

Beet pulp can be soaked without any problems. Haylage should not be soaked. A second fermentation could set in, leading to an increase of un-desirable bacteria. Because haylage already contains less WSC than hay, soaking is not necessary either.

HOW DO I KNOW IF MY HORSE IS OVERWEIGHT AND HOW MUCH?

A high BCS (see p. 52) is a clear indication that your horse is overweight.
Fat deposits can be seen, he has a cresty neck, a crease along the back,
the ribs and hip bones can no longer be felt.
The ancient creed of 'to measure is to know' applies here.
So, let's find out how much your horse weighs. Of course, a weighbridge
gives the best results, but you can also use this method:

- Measure the girth of your horse's chest just behind his forelegs.
- Measure the body length from the sternum (point of the chest) to the
  ischium (point of the buttock).
- The horse's weight is calculated by a formula that uses a constant
  which depends on the system you use, metric or imperial.
- **Metric system**: (girth squared x body length), divided by 11900
  Example: Girth 170 cm, length 210 cm
  ((170 x 170) x 210) / 11900
  This horse weighs 510 kilos.
- **Imperial system**: (girth squared x body length), divided by 330
  Example: Girth 67", length 83"
  ((67 x 67) x 83) / 330
  This horse weighs 1129 lbs.
- The formula has a margin of 10%.

Determining the weight by using a weight tape is the least accurate method.
On average it results in a weight that is 65 kilograms out (143 lbs).
Now you have to compare this with what is a normal weight for its breed.
These are roughly the weight margins for the most common breeds
(in kilos, Lbs in brackets):

- Miniature horse: 100 - 200 (220 - 440)
- Shetland pony: 150 - 250 (330 - 550)
- Welsh, Exmoor, New Forest pony: 250 - 400 (220 - 440)
- Icelandic: 300 - 450 (660 - 990)
- Arabian: 400 - 500 (880 - 1100)
- Fjord, Haflinger: 450 - 600 (990 - 1320)
- Warmblood: 500 - 700 (1100 - 1540)
- Frisian, Irish cob: 500 - 800 (1100 - 1760)
- Draught horse: 700 and heavier (1540 and up)

HOW DO I MAKE MY HORSE LOSE WEIGHT?

Provide coarse roughage with few non-structural carbohydrates and plenty of dietary fibre. Restrict grazing (see the question 'How do I make sure my horse doesn't eat too much?' on page 97). In case grazing restrictions are difficult to maintain, it might be better to take the horse off the pasture altogether. Especially EMS and PPID horses are often better off on a hay only diet.

To determine how much hay to feed, 1.5% of how much your horse has to weigh is a good amount to start with in the first month. After that, the daily ration can be lowered to 1% of the target weight. An overweight horse with a 500 kg (1100 lbs) target weight is fed 7.5 kg (16.5 lbs) of hay the first month and 5 kg (11 lbs) of hay in the following months.

Make the horse move more. This is so important that you have to call in help if you cannot take care of it yourself. Even if the horse doesn't lose weight, exercise will improve insulin sensitivity. Only give exercise if your horse can handle it, on properly trimmed hooves and preferably on hoof boots with soft insoles.

This all sounds nice and simple. In reality, unfortunately, it often turns out to be a little more difficult. To make a horse lose weight takes effort and time. Especially if your horse has to lose a lot of weight, it is best to ask a nutritionist for advice. They can explain everything about your horse's ideal target weight, its energy balance, any dietary supplements and which types of hay are good and which are not.

HOW DO I EXERCISE MY HORSE IN A RESPONSIBLE WAY?

You can start encouraging your horse to move from Obel 1, or when the horse starts to move noticeably better after one minute of walking with hoof boots and insoles, by:
- Hand walking
- Groundwork or games
- Offering social interaction with other horses

- Creating several locations with hay, water and salt licks at a fair distance from each other
- Fencing off a track in the meadow or riding arena
- Creating a paddock paradise

WHAT IS A GRAZING MUZZLE?

Grass leaf tips contain lower NSC levels. A grazing muzzle attached to the halter helps prevent the horse from grazing the grass lower down. Grazing speed decreases and food enters the digestive tract more slowly and steadily. In this way the digestion can take place more slowly and effectively. There will be fewer peaks in blood sugar levels. Less undigested carbs go from the small intestine to the large intestine. What's more, your horse can stay out on pasture longer and therefore will get more exercise.

WHAT DRUGS ARE AVAILABLE FOR LAMINITIS?

It sounds a bit bland, but there are no drugs for laminitis because it is not a disease (see the question 'Is laminitis a hoof disease?' on page 17). However, the vet can pull out a whole arsenal of drugs to help cure the underlying problems, inhibit the development of laminitis or treat complications. It is beyond the scope of this book to go into this in depth. If you want to know a lot more about it, consider reading the book 'Laminitis: understanding, cure, prevention'. We will briefly discuss a few types of medication here.

PAIN-RELIEVING AND ANTI-INFLAMMATORY DRUGS

Most pain-relieving drugs (analgesics) are also anti-inflammatory. They are NSAIDs (Non-Steroid Anti-Inflammatory Drugs). A well-known drug is phenylbutazone ('bute' or equipalazone). The inflammation that the veterinarian wants to fight is that of the dermal lamellae.

ANTICOAGULANT DRUGS

The vet may prescribe an anticoagulant drug to dissolve microthromboses. These tiny blood clots may be the result of digestive problems (see p. 32), sudden food changes or toxins in the blood (p. 34). Damage to the capillaries also causes clots. A commonly used remedy is heparin.

VASODILATOR DRUGS

These drugs dilate (widen) the blood vessels and make the blood cells less likely to stick together. The ultimate goal is to reduce blood clotting. In addition, the blood pressure is slightly lowered by some of these medicines. It is not known whether this effect reaches the dermal lamellae. The best chance of this happening is if it is injected directly into a blood vessel.

ANTIDIABETIC DRUGS

In human medicine, antidiabetic (blood sugar lowering) drugs are known to be effective in the treatment of type 2 diabetes, which also have an effect in insulin resistant horses. Metformin is the most commonly used of these. We will discuss it later.

DOPAMINE-AGONISTS

In PPID there is something wrong with the nerves that produce the hormone dopamine. Dopamine-agonists bind to the dopamine receptors in the pituitary gland in the absence of dopamine that should come from these nerves. The receptors now do their work a lot better. This is how the veterinarian tries to limit the production of ACTH by the pituitary gland (see p. 34 under 'PPID'). Horses that have not had PPID for very long can benefit from the dopamine-agonist pergolide (brand names: Prascend™ and Pergoquin™). This drug cannot cure the disease, but it can slow it down and sometimes bring it to a standstill.

ARE PAINKILLERS ALWAYS A GOOD THING?

Analgesic drugs suppress the inflammatory pain. This is a disadvantage. Your horse might move more or differently than is good for him. The lamellar connection is already damaged and may deteriorate further due to overloading. These drugs are also often bad for the intestines. In particular, your horse may get stomach problems. There is a new generation of NSAIDs that cause fewer side effects (suxibuzone and firocoxib).

On the other hand, pain stimulates the production of the hormones adrenaline, norepinephrine and dopamine. This leads to an undesirable increase in blood sugar levels and constriction of blood vessels. With pain medication it is also possible to get your horse to move with caution at an earlier stage. This is beneficial for the blood circulation.

One must always choose between what is 'humane' and what is 'good' for the horse. We should not overestimate the pain-relieving effect of these types of medication either. It is a tricky choice, but you can't avoid it most of the time. It is not necessarily good or bad to use analgesic drugs. The starting point should be: don't give it, unless this would impede the healing process. Consult your vet about this topic too.

ARE ANTI-INFLAMMATORIES NECESSARY?

Inflammation hardly plays a role in hormone-related and traumatic laminitis. In some cases, the dermal lamellae become inflamed when damaged. In that case, anti-inflammatory medication falls mainly under symptom control. This in itself is not wrong. After all, the inflammatory fluid creates a swelling that contributes to the breaking of the lamellar connection. Furthermore, an inflammation leads to the formation of blood clots. In SIRS-related laminitis the body is in an inflammatory state. Anti-inflammatories then have a more important part to play in the treatment.

DO I NEED TO GIVE STOMACH LINERS?

One of the possible side effects of the first generation of NSAIDs is an ulcer. A drug that protects the stomach wall can be used to try to prevent this. This is especially recommended when using phenylbutazone ('bute'), flunixin and ketoprofen. There are also NSAIDs on the market that cause fewer side effects. Stomach problems are seen less frequently. These drugs are the earlier mentioned suxibuzone and firocoxib.

ARE ANTICOAGULANT DRUGS NECESSARY?

If you post a message on Facebook that your horse has laminitis, you will get tons of advice. Among other things, anticoagulant medication is frequently recommended. Heparin and aspirin or willow branches and turmeric, if you are not so fond of pills and powders. This is remarkable, because hormone-related laminitis does not cause clotting problems. Although there are blood clots, they are a reaction to tissue damage. Because this is the most commonly occurring form of laminitis (80%), you may wonder whether you should go straight to anticoagulant drugs. After all, there are drawbacks as well. In chronic laminitis, the coffin bone presses against the sole from the inside out. This can damage the capillaries there. Using anticoagulants could then cause haemorrhages.

In the case of SIRS-related laminitis, however, blood clots are a possible cause (see p. 22). The use of anticoagulants at an early stage can minimise the damage later on in the disease process. As far as traumatic laminitis is concerned, we do not yet know what role blood clots play. Therefore, without knowing the cause and therefore the type of laminitis, it is not possible to say whether you should use these drugs. The advice on Facebook is well-intended, but the right person to decide whether anticoagulant medication should be used is the vet.

One more thing: anticoagulant drugs are often referred to as blood thinners. By inhibiting blood coagulation, a superficial wound will indeed continue to bleed longer. This gave rise to the idea that the blood would be thinner. However, this is not the case.

WHY DOES THE VET PRESCRIBE ASPIRIN?

Aspirin is an anticoagulant drug. It only works for a short time because it is poorly absorbed by the horse's body and then breaks down quickly. Aspirin is also used as an anti-inflammatory, while it has the weakest anti-inflammatory action of all NSAIDs. Also, for fever reduction and pain relief there are better drugs available than aspirin. In the case of a coffin bone rotation or a sinker, aspirin should not be used at all. We repeat it again just to be on the safe side: the sharp edge of the coffin bone can damage the blood vessels in the solar dermis. The anticoagulant effect of aspirin could then cause considerable bruising.

CAN I ALSO GIVE MY HORSE PARACETAMOL?

Researchers assume that paracetamol can also be used as a painkiller and fever reducer in horses. Because little scientific research has been done on it yet, your vet will either not use it yet or will be very careful prescribing it. Overdose could lead to liver damage. Horses with impaired liver function should therefore certainly not be treated with paracetamol.

WHAT ARE THE SIDE EFFECTS OF PERGOLIDE?

Pergolide is difficult to dose accurately. Overdosing can easily occur. Approximately one in ten horses will lose their appetite or show signs of depression if you start with the recommended dosage. This is called the 'pergolide veil'. It is best to stop giving the drug for a few days. Then start with a lower dose. Then slowly build up again. Only do this in consultation with your veterinarian. Diarrhea, colic and aggression are also reported as side effects.

ARE THERE NO HERBAL ALTERNATIVES TO PERGOLIDE?

We hear a lot about chastetree berry (or monk's pepper) as an herb in the treatment of PPID. Scientific studies contradict each other about whether this plant is beneficial or not. Some studies show positive effects with regard to coat problems, sweating or excessive drinking and urinating. Reduction of adiposity (see p. 37) is also mentioned. Other studies show that these positive effects do not exist. Some horse owners swear by them, others see no effect at all. Whoever is right, chastetree berry will certainly not lower the levels of ACTH in the blood. A lower risk of laminitis has also not yet been conclusively demonstrated. Therefore, this plant is not a serious alternative to pergolide.

MY VETERINARIAN MENTIONED METFORMIN. WHAT IS THAT?

This medicine inhibits, among other things, the absorption of sugar in the small intestine, as a result of which the blood sugar level goes down. This is good for horses with hormonal problems. However, the sugar now passes through to the large intestine. We do not yet know exactly what the effect of this is. It may well be that acidification and bacterial death now occur, as described on page 32 under 'Digestive problems'. If your horse now has to deal with SIRS-related laminitis, he would be jumping out of the frying pan and into the fire. Fortunately, veterinarians are reluctant to use metformin. They will emphasize the importance of weight loss, dietary changes and exercise.

MY HORSE'S HOOVES HAVE TO BE CASTED. WHAT DOES THAT MEAN?

In the acute phase, or in case of a sinker, the hoof may be casted with plaster or synthetic casting material. Sole supporting materials are sometimes included within the cast. By casting, the veterinarian or hoof care provider tries to improve the distribution of forces in the hoof, reduce sensitivity or prevent further coffin bone rotation.

Casting should be done by someone who has a great deal of experience in this area. After all, there are quite a few disadvantages. The hoof mechanism is limited. Incorrectly applied casts can pinch off the blood supply. Some materials used for fixation are not breathable. This can cause mould formation. There is also a risk of skin infection.

WHAT IS A TENOTOMY?

In a tenotomy the veterinary surgeon cuts through the deep digital flexor tendon. He does this procedure to take away the tensile force of the tendon in order to eliminate the coffin bone rotation. This surgical intervention is often undertaken despite the fact this tensile force is not the problem. The rotation of the coffin bone is caused by the inability of the lamellae, along with the extensor tendon, to offer counter force.

Usually this method is applied in a very late stage of laminitis, and mostly just to prolong the life of the horse. Whether this outweighs the list of possible complications is questionable. Swelling, pain, inflammation, connective tissue overgrowth, osteoarthritis, joint deformities and permanent tendon contraction may occur as complications. Long and intensive after-care is required.

WHAT IS A RESECTION?

With a resection, part of the hoof wall is removed. The farrier does this primarily to remove pressure and improve blood circulation. By doing so, they aim to promote better hoof growth. This should only be done if the veterinarian or the farrier at a clinic really doesn't see any other possibility. The risk of inflammation, abscesses or tissue overgrowth is present. Too much pressure is also exerted on the rest of the hoof wall after resection. If the lamellar connection all around the hoof is poor, the problem will just shift. The risk of coffin bone rotation or sinking increases. In most cases, removing pressure and improving blood circulation can also be done by bevelling the toe when trimming and using hoof boots.

SHOULD I GIVE SUPPLEMENTS?

To support the healing or to prevent a new episode of laminitis, it can be useful to use supplements. A huge range of supplements is available. The utility and necessity of some of those is questionable. It is not even known whether certain substances have an opposite effect. Supplements to promote hoof growth are not important in the early stages of laminitis.

Before you start giving supplements, you need to know which vitamins and minerals your horse is lacking. A blood test can help, although it is not always 100% reliable. Important additional information can be obtained from a nutritional analysis. If you know what your horse is taking in too little of through his feed, you know what you need to supplement. Slightly less accurate is using average values of the roughage. Due to the broad margins of minerals, you will not easily overdose.

You should know that a large surplus of certain vitamins or minerals can be just as harmful as a deficit. Do not give supplements if it is not clear that the horse is really lacking them. Do not experiment with supplements yourself, but make use of the knowledge, understanding and experience of a veterinarian or nutritionist.

DO I GIVE MAGNESIUM?

Magnesium improves the sensitivity of the body's cells to insulin. At least, that is what we assume. In humans and rats this has been demonstrated, but not yet in horses. There is even research showing that it is not. However, there is so much anecdotal evidence that it is a good idea to give your laminitic horse magnesium. Of course, this is only the case if he is really insulin-resistant.

As a first aid measure you could give magnesium even if you do not yet know the cause of the laminitis. If later it turns out that your horse is not insulin-resistant, then giving magnesium is not bad for the horse, unless he has kidney problems. If it turns out to be SIRS-related or traumatic laminitis, you simply don't give it anymore.

WHAT KIND OF MAGNESIUM SHOULD I GIVE THEN?

There are various magnesium compounds. Magnesium chelate and magnesium citrate are best absorbed by the horse's body. Magnesium oxide is cheap, but is poorly absorbed and has a laxative effect. Other compounds contain very little magnesium, are even more poorly absorbed or can cause nerve damage.

SHOULD I GIVE COPPER, ZINC OR MANGANESE?

The ideal ratio of iron, copper, zinc and manganese is 4:1:3:3. If this balance is disturbed, problems such as inexplicable laminitis, recurring abscesses, thrush and thin soles can occur. Do not blindly supplement these minerals. If you give too much of one of them, things will go even more out of balance. Ask a nutritionist for advice.

WHAT IS SUPPLEMENT X?

There are many compound supplements and vitamin and mineral balancers on the market today. They are intended to replenish nutrients or you ought to give them to increase insulin sensitivity, reduce blood sugar levels, inhibit inflammation or promote circulation. Ingredients often found in these products are:

- Minerals: magnesium, copper, zinc, manganese, sulphur, selenium
- Vitamins: A, B (especially B1), D, E and H/biotin
- Amino and fatty acids: methionine and lysine, omega-3
- Herbs: devil's claw, fenugreek, ginkgo biloba, garlic, turmeric, jiaogulan, rosehip

Of all these substances and plants, research data exists that prove or assume that they can be beneficial for horses suffering from laminitis, EMS or PPID. Whether they do so in this composition, amount and administered this way often remains the question, as there is a lot of anecdotal evidence. Whether this one pot or sachet that you have in mind can help your horse is not easy to say. It depends, among other things, on what the underlying cause is and what kind of laminitis your horse has (hormone-related, SIRS-related, traumatic). It is generally safe to try these remedies. If you have any doubts, consult a nutritionist, your vet or a phytotherapist (herbal therapist). A few tips: make sure there is no sugar in these products. Also remember that there are no panaceas that can solve laminitis or the underlying problem. And don't be tempted too much by words like 'natural', 'herbal', 'balanced' and 'complete'.

CAN I SUPPORT RECOVERY WITH HERBS?

What the previous answer said about supplements also applies to herbs. Certain plants, such as ginger, can dilute blood vessels and have an analgesic effect. Some herbs have a positive effect on insulin sensitivity and the amount of sugar in the blood. Psyllium is one such plant. Hops contain a substance that could help prevent the rapid division of bacteria in the colon. This makes it useful for a horse with SIRS-related laminitis. However, herbs are no more innocent than synthetic remedies. Whether the antibiotic substance is manufactured in a laboratory or extracted from a plant does not change the fact that you are giving antibiotics. Dosing is also a tricky issue in phytotherapy. You cannot be sure how much of the active substance is in the plant. Moreover, there are always other substances in a plant that you will inadvertently administer. There may also be an interaction with chemical drugs given to your horse. So do not go wild with plants and herbs yourself, but ask your vet or a phytotherapist for advice.

SHOULD I GIVE BIOTIN?

Biotin is often used to promote hoof growth. Firstly, accelerated hoof growth is not important in the case of laminitis. Secondly, horses make their own biotin in the intestines and they extract it from grass. You should be cautious with grass when your horse is laminitic, but it is unlikely that he will develop a biotin deficiency straight away. So just leave the biotin in the shop for a while.

WHAT ARE OMEGA FATTY ACIDS AND DO I NEED TO GIVE THEM TO MY HORSE?

Both blood clots and insulin resistance are reduced by omega-3 fatty acids. They also lower the blood pressure a little, which mean a slightly lower circulation. The supply of enzymes that break down proteins in the basal membrane also goes down as a result, which is good for horses with SIRS-related laminitis. The fatty acids also limit the production of one of these enzymes. At the same time they ensure that the blood vessels constrict less. Because of this, the blood circulation rises again.

Omega-3 retrieves the horse from green grass. In the winter or when you let your horse graze less, linseed is a good source of omega-3 fatty acids. Supplementation is usually not necessary.

ARE WILLOW BRANCHES ANY GOOD?

Willow branches contain salicin. This is the same substance found in aspirin. Horse owners give willow branches because salicin is an anti-coagulant, an anti-inflammatory and because it reduces fever and pain. In addition to the disadvantages described on page 69, there is no way of knowing how much salicin the branches contain and how much the horse eats of it. Salicin is bad for the stomach. Also remember that clotting problems do not play an important role in more than 80% of laminitis cases. You can give willow branches, but don't expect miracles. Keep an eye on how much your horse eats of it and don't give it in case of a coffin bone rotation or sinker.

WHAT IS DEVIL'S CLAW?

Devil's claw is an herbal alternative to NSAIDs. We are not yet sure about adverse effects on the stomach when used long-term. Don't give products containing devil's claw to pregnant mares. It could cause a miscarriage.

DO PROBIOTICS MAKE SENSE?

To give probiotics is to artificially, orally add bacteria to the digestive tract. You can do this to improve the pH level (acidity) and the bacterial system in the intestines. It has to be said, however, that although promising results have been achieved in test tubes, the health benefits in real horses are still difficult to prove. It remains to be seen, for example, whether the bacteria actually reach the intestines and are not broken down earlier in the digestive system. Probiotics have hardly any side effects, are easy to administer and cost little. Partly because of this, they are increasingly used in the fight against SIRS-related laminitis. With the other two forms of laminitis it makes no sense to give them.

APPLE CIDER VINEGAR IS SAID TO BE BENEFICIAL FOR MY INSULIN-RESISTANT HORSE. IS THAT TRUE?

Some studies have looked at the relationship between apple cider vinegar and blood sugar. These studies were carried out on two small groups of horses and the results are very different. A study in rats showed that cider vinegar lowers the average blood sugar level, but rats are not horses. Other studies were aimed at lowering blood sugar levels after meals. The results of these studies are of little use to us because horses should not eat meals anyway. In addition, vinegar increases the acidity of the intestines, resulting in acidification. This is precisely what we want to avoid. So, use vinegar to season your salad, but do not feed it to your horse.

EVERYONE USES CBD OIL, IT SEEMS.
CAN MY HORSE BENEFIT FROM THAT?

Cannabidiol (CBD) is a substance extracted from hemp. CBD is increasingly being used therapeutically in human medicine. Horse owners now also use it for their laminitic horses because it has analgesic and anti-inflammatory properties. With CBD oil they also aim to limit the use of NSAIDs. The benefits of CBD for the treatment of EMS are said to be reduced inflammation, lower insulin resistance and improved blood sugar levels. Note: this has been observed in humans and laboratory animals. In horses, these effects have not yet been demonstrated.

Humans generally tolerate CBD oil well. Possible side effects are diarrhea and abdominal aches. It is not known whether this is also the case in horses. CBD may also interact with other medications. In humans, reduced appetite has been mentioned as a side effect. Tell your vet if you want to give CBD oil to your horse.

WHAT IS MANUAL LYMPHATIC DRAINAGE?

The lymphatic system absorbs tissue fluid and transports it back to the vascular system. It also plays an important role in the immune system and in the disposal of waste products. Manual lymphatic drainage (MLD) is a gentle massage technique that stimulates the lymphatic system. Research shows that the application of MLD in the acute phase of laminitis can contribute to faster recovery and less damage to tissues in the hoof. This is because substances involved in inflammation are removed more quickly. Substances that reduce insulin sensitivity are also removed more quickly. This is a positive thing for horses with EMS. More good news for these horses is that MLD improves the sugar metabolism. Manual lymphatic drainage lowers blood pressure and reduces the accumulation of tissue fluid (oedema), which reduces the pressure in the hoof capsule. The blood circulation improves and the pain decreases.

IS ACUPUNCTURE HELPFUL?

In acupuncture, small needles are inserted into the body to act on blockages in energy pathways (meridians). It could enhance the positive effects of conventional treatment and reduce its side effects. One reason for this is that it releases analgesic endorphins into the body. It should also improve circulation and reduce oedema. Whether or not it works does not detract from the fact that neither the meridians nor the supposed energy flowing through them have ever been demonstrated in horses. It is also interesting to know that research has been done in humans that showed that the increased production of endorphins was independent of the place on the body where the needle was inserted. Treatment on the meridians did not yield better results. The researchers believe that the endorphin peak is a reaction to the pain caused by the needle.

The scientific journal 'Journal of Veterinary Internal Medicine' concluded in 2006 that there is no convincing evidence to recommend nor reject acupuncture in domesticated animals. Thus, after numerous studies, there is still no conclusive evidence for the effectiveness of acupuncture, but neither is there any conclusive evidence against it. You might consider it as a supportive therapy. If you use it as a substitute for regular treatment, you take the risk that your horse will not receive the care it needs.

WILL BIO-RESONANCE HELP?

Bio-resonance is a pseudo-scientific theory based on unproven assumptions that conflict with all our biological and physiological knowledge. There are some small-scale studies that are rather lame in terms of study design, which show some effect. If those studies are carried out again, but methodologically correctly, the effect cannot be demonstrated again. True, it looks impressive when machines are brought out to measure or influence vibrations and the electromagnetism of organs. However, the chance of them helping your horse is minimal. In fact, they could make the situation worse. Especially when bio-resonance is used as a diagnostic tool. Suppose the result is: 'your horse does not have insulin resistance', whereas it actually does. There is a good chance that your horse will then not receive the treatment it needs. And if the measurement wrongly shows that your horse does suffer from an ailment, the risk of over-treatment is imminent. You could simply start a treatment that your horse does not need.

HOW ABOUT HOMEOPATHY?

Homeopathy uses extremely low concentrations of substances to solve problems that they could cause if taken in higher concentrations. The concentrations are even that low that the substance is no longer detectable in the remedy. Theories as to how it would still work mention a never proven form of memory that water would have.

There is no convincing scientific evidence that homeopathy works. There are studies which show that homeopathy is effective in certain human conditions; there are also studies which show that it does not work at all. Studies on its efficacy in animals are scarce and the results are not strong. One of the major problems is that the scientific standard of double-blind randomised trials with a control group is difficult to carry out. Homeopathy is said to treat the patient, not the disease. The patient's entire medical background plays a role in this. No two cases are the same. As a result, the individuals in the study population cannot be randomly assigned to groups (those who receive the treatment, those who receive a placebo and those who are in the control group and receive nothing). Also, horses have often had different owners. Their medical history is therefore not always available.

If you are comfortable with the fact that no one can prove to you how the treatment works, you can try homeopathy. It is completely safe and has no side effects. Replacing a proven therapy with homeopathy is not as good an idea. Don't lose sight of reality either. If your horse is severely insulin resistant, you really need to change its diet and exercise, and you shouldn't rely on homeopathy.

CAN I USE MAGNETIC BANDAGES TO IMPROVE BLOOD CIRCULATION?

A highly concentrated salt solution can be put into a thin glass tube and then made to move by a strong magnet. To conclude that this will also be the case with blood in a flexible blood vessel under the influence of a weak magnet is a bridge too far. Fortunately, the researcher did not do so in this example. Unfortunately, the manufacturers of magnetic bandages cut some corners and claim that their product will dramatically increase blood flow. If it were the case that a magnet stimulates the blood flow, you would expect the skin to become red and warm underneath the magnet. This is difficult to determine in a horse's hoof, but it is certainly not the case in a human hand. And wouldn't the magnetic field of an MRI scanner, that is thousands of times stronger, make you explode? Well, luckily that is not the case. There are heaps of scientific publications that show that magnets do not have a positive influence on blood flow. There is also no convincing scientific evidence of positive effects such as removing toxins, reducing inflammation and pain or healing of damaged tissue, which manufacturers and magnetic therapists refer to. For the time being, we assume that it is mainly the placebo effect that does its job well. On page 82 you can read whether this effect also exists in horses.

WHAT IS DETOXIFICATION AND IS IT NECESSARY?

Detoxification - also known as detox, cleansing or drainage - is the removal of waste products and toxins from the body. On page 34 you have read which toxins can 'contaminate' the horse's body. Many of them are easy to remove by feeding your horse differently or being cautious with medication, vaccinations or deworming. For example, you can opt to worm only if a real worm infection has been demonstrated through manure testing. In fact, research shows that 80% of horses are unnecessarily dewormed. Toxins as a result of chronic kidney or liver problems, blood poisoning or Monday disease require treatment of these primary problems.

Detox remedies with green clay, chlorophyll or certain minerals (especially silicic acid) would be supportive. However, there is no scientific evidence for this. The best way to get rid of toxins is still to rely on a properly functioning liver, kidneys, urinary tract and intestines. By exercise, by offering high-fibre food to the intestines and, of course, by ensuring that no new toxins are added and that the amount of waste products remains low.

THERE IS SOME REVOLUTIONARY ALTERNATIVE THERAPY OR A NEW DRUG. IS IT WORTH TRYING?

Not every horse heals equally well and quickly from laminitis. Therapies, drugs, dietary changes, modifications in housing, exercise and hoof maintenance are sometimes unsuccessful. When you then read about a new miracle cure or a great new therapy, the temptation is great to pin your hopes on it. However, you should be careful with this. Sometimes they are based on assumptions or unproven theories. You should also remember that anecdotal evidence is no evidence. Another thing is that science sometimes discovers a property of a certain substance that could be of benefit to laminitic horses. This is then taken out of context on internet forums and social media. People enthusiastically start fiddling around with plants that contain that substance. Nevertheless, it is better to wait and carefully follow scientific developments until a substance has proven to be effective, useful and safe.

Have a good talk with your vet, your hoof care provider or a nutritionist. Voice your concerns. Critically reassess together whether all the conditions for a reasonable chance of recovery have been met. It may well be that someone has overlooked something. You can always ask for a second opinion from another vet.

If you do choose the new therapy or remedy, be sure to look closely at the theory behind it. Do not take things at face value just because they are on the internet. Look up information, ask the opinion of both those in favour and those against. Preferably these are people who are professionally involved. Also make sure that it does not interfere with the other aspects of treatment. Some substances can have a negative interaction with certain medications. Side effects are not always known for brand-new drugs. They may do more harm to the horse than bring relief. Also watch out for 'two captains on one ship'. If different people treating your horse are giving contradictory advice, it will certainly not help the healing process. Tell everyone concerned with your horse's treatment that you are going down this road.

WHAT IS THE PLACEBO EFFECT AND DOES IT ALSO EXIST IN HORSES?

In 1971, a study was conducted on treating a herpes virus with fluorescent light. The researchers reported a significant improvement in 87% of the participants. Later research showed that this method could by no means have been effective. We now attribute the impressive positive outcome of this study to the placebo effect. This is when we see an improvement after using a drug or therapy without them actually being able to cause the improvement. The placebo effect is due to the expectation or hope that they do. It is also possible that the improvement does take place, but that this would also have been the case if the remedy or therapy had not been used.

Of course, a horse does not know what to expect. Therefore, the placebo effect does not actually play a role for the horse itself. The owner and the therapist, on the other hand, do have their expectations and hopes. Especially for you as a horse owner, it is difficult to withdraw from this, especially if the reputation or the persuasiveness of the practitioner is high. Another problem is that we tend to think that when two things succeed each other, the second is caused by the first. If the first was even intended to make the second happen, the placebo effect is lurking. Clean a gemstone in a mountain stream and place it on your horse's third chakra. If his blood sugar is better the next day, it must be thanks to this treatment, right?

TREATMENT X WORKS VERY WELL FOR MY HORSE.
ISN'T THAT PROOF THAT TREATMENT X WORKS?

You have already seen the term 'anecdotal evidence' used a few times, but what is it? Anecdotal evidence is non-scientific evidence that is based on some (or a lot of) people's experiences. In the case of treatment with a substance or a therapy, we could call it 'happy customer proof'. However, to demonstrate whether a treatment works or not, these experiences are rather useless. You are never unbiased and that can easily be explained:

- No one can escape the placebo effect. Certainly not if you have already invested a lot of time, money and effort in a treatment method. Then you want to see improvement so much that it will take place. Or so it seems.

- You cannot estimate whether the health of your horse would have improved without the treatment. We usually focus on several problems at the same time. Is the improvement in your horse's insulin resistance due to treatment X or did the new batch of hay that contains less sugar did the trick?
- The manifestations of a disease can fluctuate. The seasonal rise in ACTH in a horse with PPID (see p. 41) is a good example of this. If at the end of this period you have treated your horse with remedy X, you can be mistaken and think that remedy X is to be thanked for the improvement in clinical presentation.
- It is difficult to tell the difference between suppressed clinical signs and an actual cure. Less pain does not necessarily mean that the source of the pain has been removed.
- You don't want to disappoint the practitioner. As crazy as it sounds, we have that tendency. If the practitioner thinks to be successful when this is not actually the case, one has to be very confident to go against it.

Treatments that are truly successful provide tons of anecdotal evidence of course. But that evidence is in addition to clinical experience from veterinarians and evidence from solid scientific research. So, don't blindly follow your friend at the stable who won't stop raving about treatment X because it saved her horse from death. Maybe it did so; maybe not.

TREATMENT X IS CLEARLY WORKING FOR MY FRIEND'S HORSE BUT NOT FOR MINE. HOW IS THAT POSSIBLE?

We never treat just one aspect of the horse or its condition. The horse's body is a complex framework in which all kinds of systems work closely together and influence each other. Intestines, blood vessels, hormonal glands, nerves … it's all connected. Perhaps the treatment of your friend's horse affects another aspect of the disease a bit more. Do you know all the ins and outs of nutrition, housing, exercise and hoof care that her horse receives? Is her horse of the same breed, the same sex, the same age as yours? Does her horse have the same underlying causes? Are we talking about the same type (hormone-related, SIRS-related, traumatic) of laminitis? After having read the answer to the previous question, you may even wonder if the treatment her horse is getting really works as well as you think.

You could ask your friend to tell you what else she's doing to help her horse. Also, ask the person who treats her horse why the same treatment turns out to be less successful for your horse. Maybe they see a difference you don't see. If you have not already done so: find the cause, together with your vet and remove it as much as possible. Make sure that the hooves are properly and regularly trimmed and look into the benefits of hoof boots. Make an effort to improve every aspect of the living conditions of your horse. Who knows, maybe your horse will soon be doing so well that your friend will wonder how on earth that is possible.

SOMEONE OFFERS DISTANT HEALING OF MY HORSE. SHOULD I ACCEPT THIS OFFER?

There are people who claim they can transcend the limitations of distance in space or time when treating a horse. However, as yet, there is no scientific reason to have confidence in the clinical efficacy of 'distant healing' (or for 'nearby healing', for that matter). In this form of interaction with the patient, the expectation and belief of the recipient is often seen as an indispensable part of the treatment. This makes double-blind trials with control group impossible by definition. This is in addition to the fact that we would then have to answer the question whether horses have expectations and beliefs. Healers then say that modern research methods, techniques and instruments are not capable of properly investigating healing and should therefore be adapted. In doing so, they place themselves outside the scientific model of thought. A critical look at healing is thus off the table and science gets the blame.

Healers also tend to cite their own successes as proof, while their failures are never mentioned and quickly forgotten. There is also no way to prove whether the success is really theirs. Any criticism is dismissed with the reproach that people are not open to it and that 'there is more between heaven and earth'. The supporters simply declare that they do believe it exists or even that they know it exists, followed by just another spectacular anecdote.

As it stands, there is an unacceptable risk that your horse will not get the treatment he needs if you replace any part of it with remote healing. The only benefit may be that adding healing to the treatment may increase your own motivation and perseverance in the fight against laminitis. But to pay someone who lives miles away to do so, ...

THE VET, THE HOOF CARE PROVIDER, MY FRIENDS AT THE STABLE AND THE WHOLE OF FACEBOOK SAY SOMETHING ELSE. WHO SHOULD I BELIEVE?

It is good that there is so much information available and that we can exchange ideas with so many people. The downside, however, is that this can lead to contradictory and sometimes downright wrong advice. This is partly because the three different forms of laminitis are often lumped together. Non-professionals and fellow horse owners are particularly prone to this. For example, as soon as you drop the L-word, magnesium is referred to as a panacea, even though your horse has SIRS-related laminitis following a persistent inflammation. Magnesium will do nothing for that. The focus on anti-coagulants and anti-inflammatories for hormone-related laminitis is also one such example. With the best of intentions, people give advice without knowing the underlying cause. They have never seen the horse, do not know its medical history, and do not know what you have already done to improve its living conditions. When you give them this information, they either read over it in their enthusiasm or they see it too much through the lenses of their own experience. Garlic saved their horse from certain death, so every horse that suffers from laminitis should be put on garlic immediately.

The attention and involvement of facebook users and your riding buddies give you support in these difficult times when your horse is sick and in pain. That is very important. Moreover, different experiences can bring you ideas that you might not have thought of. However, it is advisable to use the knowledge and experience of professionals in the first place. The vet is the right person to turn to for diagnosis and medical treatment; the hoof care provider knows all about your horse's hooves; a nutritionist can help you if your horse needs to lose weight or if supplements need to be given.

Unfortunately, there can also be differences of opinion between them. The saying 'cobbler, stick to your last' still applies here. If you have a good hoof care provider, trust that they know better than the vet how to trim the hooves. But don't let the hoof care provider interpret X-rays or blood values. Of course, it works best if everyone who looks after your horse professionally is more or less on the same page. In the best case, they treat your horse in a multidisciplinary way and consult with each other. If there are too many differences between how they want to do things, discuss it with them. If you cannot work it out, it is best to find another professional to replace one of them.

BUT WHAT IF A PROFESSIONAL IS TALKING NONSENSE?

We all know the example of a vet who strongly recommended that a horse be put to sleep, which fortunately was not heeded. Years later, the horse is still happily trotting through the meadow in perfect health. The farrier who claimed that you would drive your horse to its death if you removed the therapeutic shoes. If only they could see your horse galloping down the gravel path today. Just because someone has been in a profession for many years does not mean that they are always right. They may have developed a blind spot for certain solutions or they may not have kept up with the latest insights in their field for some time. Convenience can also slip in. In that case, you are offered standard solutions. Horse with a cresty neck? Must be laminitic or else it will be soon. NSAIDs, stable rest and a pair of shoes will do the trick. Or perhaps someone is strongly convinced of a particular approach. A hoof care provider with 20 years' experience will never recommend therapeutic shoes; their fellow farrier hardly knows how to spell 'hoof boot'.

Don't hold it against any of them, just make sure you get the right people for your horse. Right in the sense of experienced, knowledgeable, modern, curious and flexible. A civilised sized ego is also a plus. Now the opinions and experiences of the members of your favourite facebook groups and your riding buddies will come in handy. Ask them to also back up their opinions. Once you have brought in the right experts, there is little left for you to do to get the best out of everyone. Your horse will be very grateful.

HOW LONG DOES IT TAKE FOR LAMINITIS TO CURE?

Each horse has a different tolerance for pain, a different reaction to chang-
ing circumstances and a different self-healing capacity. It is therefore difficult to predict how recovery will take place, but let us give it a try. How long
it takes for your horse to recover depends largely on how bad the laminitis
was in the first place and how quickly you were able to remove the cause
and start the treatment. A good vet and hoof care provider will make sure
that it does not last any longer than is strictly necessary. Finally, your own
role is very important. Have you been able to perfect your horse's living
conditions? Adaptations in diet, housing and exercise are indispensable for
a good and successful recovery of the laminitic patient. If all this is in order,
a horse that has become laminitic for the first time, where the cause was an
external incident (i.e. not a hormonal disorder or chronic inflammation) and
where that cause was quickly remedied and there is no coffin bone rotation
or damage to the hoof capsule, will normally be cured within six to twelve
weeks. After that, it takes about a year for the damage to the hoof tissue to
grow out (see the question 'What is a laminitic ring?' on page 25).

In the case of a coffin bone rotation, a sinker, or severe damage to tissues such as the coffin bone, it takes much longer. The damage may be so
extensive as to be irreversible. A horse in which the coffin bone is largely
demineralised (osteoporosis) will always remain laminitic to a greater or
lesser extent. As long as the cause is not under control, there is a good
chance that your horse will remain laminitic or will repeatedly become
so. The same applies if the living conditions do not improve. If your horse
does not get proper, natural exercise, spends its days in a box and is
fed high-sugar grass, pellets or grains, it will take a very long time for a
well-intentioned painkiller or anti-inflammatory to work. Also, if the hoof
care is poor or old-fashioned, you might have to wait for things to improve
for a long time. Hoof boots, on the other hand, are very helpful in speed-
ing up healing. From page 113 onwards, we go into detail about hoof care
and protection.

In some cases, the underlying condition is incurable or you can't get a grip on it. Some horses with EMS or PPID remain laminitic for the rest of their lives. They have better periods and lesser periods. Your job then is to limit the damage and treat complications such as abscesses. Not a pleasant prospect, but a rewarding and noble job.

HOW WILL I KNOW WHEN LAMINITIS IS OVER?

The first indication that the acute phase of laminitis might be over is when you no longer see the clinical signs described on page 50. Obel 0 (p. 53) is also good news, of course. Your hoof care provider will notice things that you might not. If you have any doubts, ask them if they think the worst is over. If you really want to be sure, your vet can perform a clinical examination again. Blood test results and X-rays are very enlightening. The latter in particular show when chronic laminitis is no longer present. Your vet can also tell you whether your horse really is no longer laminitic or whether it is only the clinical signs that have been successfully suppressed. The amount of pain, for example, is not the best indicator of the horse's condition. Some horses do not show signs of pain any more while there is still tissue damage.

HOW DO I PICK UP MY HORSE'S TRAINING AGAIN?

OK, those hooves look fine again. Saddle up and ride. Well, no. Laminitis is not a hoof disease, remember? There is always more to it than that. It takes time before everything is back to normal. The laminitis has weakened the hoof, and it takes a while to recover from that weakness. Be patient and let the hoof settle down before you put your horse back to work. The same goes for the underlying ailments. They may not be so serious as to make your horse laminitic, but it may well be that your horse is still recovering from, for example, an infection. Ask your vet about the status of that.

If you are planning to start working with your horse again, do it for him and not for yourself. Do not ride your horse at first. Take your horse out on nice little walks with well-trimmed hooves in hoof boots. You can also exercise the horse by doing ground work or through horseplay. Offer social interaction with other horses, Place hay feeders, water and salt lick as far apart as possible. This will keep the horse moving. Maybe you could fence off a track in the pasture or arena. A paddock paradise, as described on page 107, also stimulates movement very well.

If you are going to ride again, only do so when all movement is problem-free (Obel 0), on hoof boots with insoles and when the sole of the hoof itself is thick enough. Your hoof care provider can tell you when they think this is the case. The veterinarian can determine sole thickness more accurately with an X-ray. Gradually increase the training in length and intensity. Don't make the distances too long, don't over ask the horse and ride at a slow to medium pace. Let the horse decide for itself where to put its hooves. Lunging and exercising in a horse walker will put too much strain on the recovering hooves. Do not do this for the time being.

HOW DO I PREVENT MY HORSE FROM GETTING LAMINITIS AGAIN?

In the chapter 'Causes', you have read about all the different things that can lead to laminitis. Unfortunately, it is not possible to recognise all these causes and then keep them under control all the time. Moreover, some underlying ailments can be incurable. Sooner or later, this will lead to such a high risk of laminitis that a small push is enough to start the misery. If your horse has become laminitic despite all the precautions and good care, then you will need to prevent it from worsening. So, it is better to let go of the idea that laminitis can always be prevented.

Nevertheless, we must try to keep the risk as low as possible. Horses that have had laminitis before run a greater risk of being struck again. This is, among other things, because they are more likely to have painful hooves due to damaged tissues. Pain makes the blood sugar level rise and narrows the blood vessels. But much more often it is because the causes have not all disappeared completely.

Actually, prevention is not much different than treatment:
- Step 1: make sure the cause is and remains gone or is as much as possible under control
- Step 2: ensure that the hooves get properly and regularly trimmed
- Step 3: optimise the living conditions nutrition, housing and exercise

Most horses get laminitis again because attention to these points slackens as soon as the horse is doing better.

WHEN DO I KNOW THAT EUTHANASIA IS THE ONLY OPTION LEFT?

Some horse owners will at some point have to consider whether it is still justifiable to keep their horse alive. Horses that have been stumbling through the pasture with perforated soles for a long time with no prospect of recovery and are in terrible pain every day and cannot tell you that it has been enough. The responsibility for deciding on euthanasia therefore always lies with you, the owner. Although the final decision is yours, the veterinarian is in the best position to make objective judgements about your horse's well-being now and in the future. They can compare your horse's situation with other horses they have had in their practice. There is also no emotional tie that prevents them from forming a neutral opinion. A good vet will look again at the causes, the degree of lameness, the seriousness of the complications and to what extent the treatment is effective. The success of pain relief is very important to them. They will often consult with your horse's other caregivers, such as the hoof care provider.

The vet is objective enough to also see to what extent you are able to provide the care that is needed. If, for whatever reason, you cannot provide that care, it is not fair to let your horse suffer. It is up to you to decide what the outcome will be. It is a difficult decision that often takes more time with the owner than the vet thinks is desirable from the horse's interest. Fortunately, they know that this is part of their job. They will give you time to think about their advice. During this process, you should not hesitate to ask them to explain their advice again if necessary. You can also ask for the opinion of another vet. If you really cannot let go of your horse yet, then terminal or palliative care may still be an option. Whether you will be doing your horse a favour this way, is another matter.

NUTRITION

WHAT IS THE BEST DIET FOR MY LAMINITIC HORSE?

In the previous chapter, you read about soaked hay and magnesium as an emergency diet in case of acute laminitis. With that, we are trying to tackle insulin issues. If your horse is not in the 80% of cases where insulin resistance is the main problem, then being fed this way will not be harmful. However, be careful not to supplement magnesium to horses with kidney problems.

Now that you have a better grip of the laminitis, let's have a look at what your horse can best eat from now on. Give high-fibre, coarse-stem hay with less than 10% ESC, starch and fructan (see the question 'There's not just one kind of sugar, is there?' on page 38). If it is above 10%, you can soak the hay (see p. 61). Preferably choose lucerne (alfalfa) hay (contains a lot of magnesium) with few leaves and mostly stems. Lucerne hay can be high in proteins. There are horses that react badly to it. Probably they convert proteins into sugar very effectively. A high dry matter content in roughage is also good. You can have your forage tested for energy, sugars, protein and dry matter content. You can also have an extensive analysis done. This is quite a bit more expensive, but it will give you a good picture of all the important minerals and trace elements. With this information, a nutritionist can very specifically recommend supplements. Until then, you can give a broad-spectrum supplement (balancer). This provides the most important vitamins and minerals.

Of course, always provide clean drinking water and a regular salt lick. If you give your horse a balancer, make sure that the salt lick really only contains salt and no extra minerals or trace elements. You don't want to give them twice.

CAN I STILL FEED MY HORSE PELLETS AND GRAINS?

Well, better not do that. There are too many fast sugars in this type of food and we always serve it in rations. This causes high peaks in the blood sugar levels. This is not good, because it can lead to hormone-related laminitis. When the fast carbs reach the large intestine (colon), they contribute to SIRS-related laminitis.

AND HORSE MUESLI OR PELLETS WITH EXTRA VITAMINS AND MINERALS?

That depends on which one you feed. Muesli is just a different form of the same product. Ground and pressed muesli is simply called pellets or concentrates. If it contains extra vitamins, minerals and trace elements, it is called vitaminised or enriched. There are horse mueslis without grains that remain under 10% sugar and starch. The same manufacturer may have another muesli on the market which is well over the 20% mark. So always read the labels carefully. Molasses and cereals should be avoided. Also pay attention to the amount of iron in the product. This must be as low as possible. Ideally, there should be no iron in it at all. An iron surplus is associated with insulin resistance. Also ask yourself why you want to give these products. Are you afraid that your horse will be short of something? Then it's better to give a balancer as an extra on top of the roughage. If you then have a roughage analysis carried out to see whether your horse is indeed getting too little of certain substances, you are doing it all the right way.

WHAT IS A BALANCER?

Your horse needs a minimum amount of certain minerals, vitamins and trace elements. In particular, horses that eat mainly hay or are on a weight loss diet are more likely to be deficient than horses that can graze without restriction. A broad-spectrum supplement, or with a hip word 'balancer', is intended to balance a roughage diet by supplementing the daily requirement of vitamins, minerals and trace elements. A balancer is second best to a supplement formulated by a nutritionist for your horse based on blood tests and roughage analysis. Rather, your horse should eat a varied, healthy, natural diet that contains everything.

Also read the ingredients list carefully. Some balancers contain as much as 20% sugar and starch. And again: a horse which is fed a balancer should not also get all kinds of minerals through its lick. A simple salt lick is sufficient.

WHAT DO I NEED TO PAY ATTENTION TO WHEN IT COMES TO DRINKING WATER?

Always provide fresh and clean drinking water. Algae, dead leaves, insects, manure, urine and rust in the pipes or the drinking bowl itself can contaminate the water. This can all result in toxins. Ditch water can be polluted by illegal discharges, manure and pesticides. It is possible to have your horse's drinking water analysed.

WHAT KIND OF SALT LICK DOES MY LAMINITIC HORSE NEED?

Sodium is a mineral that is difficult for a horse to obtain. Therefore, you should provide a simple salt lick. The most striking feature of a lick from the Himalayas is that it has been in a plane for a long time. It contains too little zinc, copper and manganese. Licks which taste of apple or contain molasses should also be left in the shop. The horse has to use the lick to get salt, not because it likes the taste of apples or sugar. The red coloured licks often contain too much iron. A surplus of iron contributes to the development or aggravation of insulin resistance.

HOW MUCH DOES MY HORSE NEED TO EAT?

If your horse is not overweight, you should feed it between 1.5% and 2% of its weight in roughage. So, for a 600 kg (1300 lbs) horse that is between 9 and 12 kg (29.8 - 26.4 lbs). If your horse needs to lose weight, then feed it 1.5% of its target weight. You do this for a month. After that you give 1%. If your horse is to weigh 500 kg (1100 lbs), then first give it 7.5 kg (19.5 lbs) of roughage and after that 5 kg (11 lbs).

IN FACT, MY HORSE IS TOO THIN. WHAT CAN I GIVE HIM TO SAFELY PUT ON WEIGHT?

First, you need to be sure that your horse really needs to gain weight. Many horse owners get it wrong when it comes to estimating the correct weight of their horse. If your horse has only just recovered from laminitis and the insulin problems are not yet fully under control, it is probably a good idea to keep the weight a little below its ideal level. Especially if his hooves have not yet fully recovered. Discuss this with your vet.

For a horse that needs to gain weight while it is susceptible to laminitis, the basis is also grass or roughage that is low in sugar, starch and fructan and contains a good deal of dietary fibre. You can feed beet pulp or lucerne (alfalfa) hay to add more energy (calories), while keeping the amount of fast carbohydrates down. Alternatively, you can feed high-fat feed such as linseed. Vegetable oil contains slow-release calories and is therefore recommended by some people to help your horse put on weight. Some oils, such as sunflower and maize oil, only contain the wrong amount and ratio of omega fatty acids. This will do your horse more harm than good. If you want to give oil, it is best to ask a nutritionist for help.

HIS WEIGHT IS ABSOLUTELY FINE AND YET HE STILL HAS PROBLEMS. HOW CAN THAT BE?

A correct body weight does not always mean that the nutrition is correct too. There may still be a deficiency of certain minerals and vitamins or a wrong balance between them. This could mean that your horse is unable to rid itself of its laminitis. Soil and roughage analysis can help you further. If these indicate a particular deficiency or imbalance, blood tests can confirm that your horse is actually experiencing this too. Now, a nutritionist can advise you on how to solve this problem.

WHEN IS GRASS LOW IN CARBOHYDRATES?

For horses with hormonal problems, it is mainly the fast sugars that we want to see as little of as possible in the plant. The quantities of these sugars change throughout the day and the year. This depends on the amount and strength of sunlight, the ambient temperature, the availability of water and nutrients and the growth phase the grass plant is in. Obviously, we cannot discuss here the effect of every combination of these factors on the quantity of sugars. The rule of thumb is that the sugar level in the grass is at its lowest:
- at night and in the very early morning,
- when it has not been colder than 5 °C (41 °F) at night,
- while sufficient water and nutrients were available, and
- the grass plant has mainly leaves and no heads.

During the day, sugar levels will rise. More hours of sunshine result in higher sugar content. As spring progresses, this will become more and more the case. Cloud cover and shade actually slow down the increase. Keep an eye not only on the percentages but also on the total amount of grass your horse eats. In spring, grass grows at an explosive rate. A horse that eats a lot of grass with a low percentage of ESC will still ingest too much of it.

For horses that are susceptible to SIRS-related laminitis, the fructan content needs to be low. These include horses with damage to the intestinal wall after colic or horses with a chronic inflammation somewhere in the body. Although fructan levels can also fluctuate throughout the day and change quickly, sunny mornings after a cold night are particularly dangerous. This is especially common in early spring and autumn.

The amount of fructan in grass also increases if the important growth factors of water and nutrients are not sufficiently present. After a long period of drought, for example, the number of laminitis cases increases. As you may have read earlier, grass also produces fructan as an antifreeze (see the question 'What is fructan?' on page 38). In autumn, when the night frost returns and the sun shines happily during the day, the risk of high fructan levels is greater. On average, April, May, October and November are the months when we see the highest values.

HOW USEFUL IS AN APP OR A WEBSITE THAT PREDICTS FRUCTAN LEVELS?

If we consider that at least 80% of all laminitis cases are hormone-related and fructan plays no role whatsoever in this form, it is strange that horse owners place so much trust in apps and websites that predict fructan levels. Yet these are not entirely redundant. For horses affected by SIRS-related laminitis, it is of course the fructan levels themselves that are important. For horses with hormonal problems, the usefulness of this type of warning system lies primarily in the fact that it provides a picture of how much sugar the plant contained a short time before. High fructan levels are not possible without a preceding sugar surplus (fructan is made up of sugar molecules, remember?). There is a good chance that this will recur in the short term and put your horse at risk of hormone-related laminitis.

CAN MY HORSE STILL GO OUT TO PASTURE?

That depends on his condition. A heavily insulin-resistant horse that would become laminitis, so to speak, from the smell of grass might be better off in a spacious paddock or on a track in a paddock paradise (see p. 107). You can then completely control what and how much he eats. If you eventually get the insulin resistance under control, you can carefully let him out in the field with a grazing muzzle when the grass is low on sugars. Unfortunately, for some horses with PPID and severe insulin resistance, this will never be the case.

If your horse has not had hormone-related laminitis, then it all becomes a lot easier. In the case of SIRS-related laminitis, you should still keep an eye on the fructan levels before putting him out to pasture. In all cases, it is important to wait until the hooves are healthy again before letting your horse out to graze. Do it with care and maintain grazing restrictions. The answer to the next question explains what these are.

HOW DO I MAKE SURE MY HORSE DOESN'T EAT TOO MUCH?

You can take the following measures to ensure that your horse does not eat too much or too quickly and thus takes in too many carbohydrates when grazing:

- Use a grazing muzzle. Grass leaf tips contain less sugar. A muzzle ensures that your horse does not gobble up the grass to the root. Grazing speed decreases as well. The food enters the digestive tract more slowly and more steadily. The carbohydrates are therefore better digested.
- Avoid overgrazing. Shortly gnawed grass contains a lot of carbohydrates.
- Offer strip grazing. The area to be grazed can be shifted, enlarged or reduced every day by using electric fencing and stakes.
- Divide your field into plots. Let your horse graze a plot until the grass is about 4 centimetres (1 1/2") high. Then put him in the next plot. The grazed part can now regrow.

- Hand grazing is another way to limit grazing time.
- Put a sign on the fence of the meadow explaining clearly why you do not appreciate people feeding your horse uninvited. Also put your telephone number on the sign so that well-meaning passers-by can ask you for more information.
- Horses that are susceptible to laminitis (overweight, EMS, PPID, high-risk breeds) should not be allowed to graze too much, if at all. They are better off in a paddock paradise, a riding arena or in a fenced off part of a yard.

ARE ALL GRASS TYPES EQUALLY DANGEROUS?

Some grasses contain much more non-structural carbohydrates than others. Unfortunately, lots of pastures are full of the sugar-rich species. These include English and Italian rye grass, brome grass, tall fescue and meadow fescue. If you have your own fields, you might consider reseeding them with a special horse pasture mix. This contains the seeds of creeping soft grass, meadow foxtail, orchard grass, phleum (specifically timothy grass) and red fescue. These grass types are low in sugar.

WHAT IS COW GRASS?

Much of the grassland has been cultivated for high milk or meat production. The focus is on generous levels of non-structural carbohydrates and proteins. The grass also has to start growing early in the year, last until late in the year and be able to withstand being trampled on. We call this grass cow grass. It is usually English rye grass. Full of sugars and not good for horses.

CAN MY HORSE ONLY EAT HAY NOW?

The good thing about hay is that, just like grass, you can have it tested. If it contains too many fast sugars and fructan (water-soluble carbohydrates), you can do something about it by soaking and rinsing. If you grow your own hay, you can regulate the amount of carbohydrates by choosing the right time to cut it. Otherwise, talk to your roughage supplier to see if they can supply low-sugar hay. Another advantage of hay is that you can decide how much your horse gets, when and how (hay net, slow feeder).

On the other hand, grazing is an important activity for your horse and you should not just take it away. Hopefully, you can go a long way with the grazing restriction measures described on page 97. Combine this with feeding hay to further control sugar consumption. Unfortunately, for some horses, pasture is really out of the question. Horses with severe EMS or PPID will have to make do with just hay.

IS ANY KIND OF HAY GOOD?

Grass varieties that contain a lot of sugar produce hay that contains a lot of sugar. The type of soil the grass has grown on, the fertiliser used and the time of mowing, both during the day and the year, also influence the amount of carbohydrates in the grass. What the grass looks, feels or smells like says nothing. The very best hay comes from natural species-rich grasslands on nutrient-poor soil. The grasses and herbs that are characteristic of this type of soil contain little sugar and many important nutrients. If you cannot get this type of hay, give hay from grasses that are low in sugar, grown on sensibly fertilised land and cut at a time when the sugar content was as low as possible. First-cut hay often contains a lot of non-structural carbohydrates. Second cut is a better choice, although it is usually over-fertilised. The hay should also not be too old. Unfortunately, you do not always have an influence on all these factors. That is why it is a good idea to have your hay tested, especially when you buy a large batch of hay. Knowing what you are feeding your horse is an indispensable part of your battle against laminitis, insulin resistance or obesity.

SHOULD I HAVE THE SOIL OR THE HAY ANALYSED?

We have already talked a few times about soil and roughage analysis. You can use this to find out if there is a particular shortage of nutrients or if the ratio of certain minerals is not optimal. If you know what your horse is not getting enough of through its feed, you know what you need to supplement. The amount of sugar, starch and fructan in the roughage is also important. You want to keep these as low as possible, while at the same time you want to feed your horse lots of fibre. A high dry matter content is also a good characteristic of roughage. You can have your forage tested for energy, sugars, protein and dry matter content. You can also have an extensive analysis done. This is quite a bit more expensive, but it will give you a good picture of all the important minerals and trace elements.

Furthermore, you can have a soil sample analysed. Minerals that are not present in the soil will not miraculously appear in the grass. Please note that the result of a soil analysis is not representative of the amount of minerals that will eventually be absorbed by the grass plant. However, a soil analysis is a good basis for fertilisation advice.

IS FREE CHOICE HAY ALWAYS RIGHT?

Your horse may do fine on 'all-you-can-eat', but this is not the case for every horse. For a long time, we assumed that all horses should have unlimited access to hay. If they ate too much of it at first, it would reduce by itself. No access to food would lead to stress and thus to an increased production of cortisol. The vasoconstrictive effects of this hormone, among others, contribute to the development of laminitis. Cortisol also reduces sensitivity to insulin. Today we know that this is an oversimplification of the situation. For insulin-resistant horses and horses with PPID in particular, the amount of fast sugars (the simple and double carbohydrates) and starch that they eat determines the risk of laminitis. If you feed these animals on unlimited hay without having the hay tested, then you are taking a great risk. Also, for horses with SIRS-related laminitis, unlimited hay is not a good idea by definition. Some horses overeat. Fast sugars, starch and fructan end up in the large intestine and can cause problems as described on page 32 under 'Digestive problems'.

IS A HAY NET OR SLOWFEEDER A GOOD IDEA?

Hay offered in a hay net or slow feeder requires your horse to make a greater effort to eat. As with the use of a grazing muzzle, it will eat more slowly. The carbohydrates enter the digestive tract at a slower pace and more evenly. As a result, they are better digested. The enzymes in the small intestine have time to break down the fast sugars and the starch. As a result, they do not end up in the large intestine, where they could contribute to acidification, bacterial death and, ultimately, SIRS-related laminitis. Fructan also enters the large intestine in a more measured way, so there is no or less acidification. Horses that eat more slowly are also less likely to suffer from obesity. So yes, a hay net or slow feeder is a good idea.

WHAT IS GRASS SEED HAY AND IS IT GOOD FOR MY HORSE?

Grass seed hay is a by-product of growing grass for seed. Most of the non-structural carbohydrates are in the seed which goes to the seed trade. The stalks consist mainly of dietary fibre (structural carbohydrates) and, when dried into hay, are good low-energy roughage for laminitic horses or horses that need to lose weight. Besides the fact that grass seed hay contains less energy, horses also have to chew this roughage quite a bit longer. This results in more saliva, which is good for the digestion. The structural carbohydrates ensure that the intestines have to work harder. Healthy intestines are important in the context of laminitis.

There are also disadvantages to grass seed hay. It contains fewer vitamins, minerals, trace elements and proteins than ordinary hay. A bigger problem is a symbiotic fungus (endophyte) the grass seed grass has been deliberately contaminated with in order to make the plant stronger and protect it against insect damage. Unfortunately, this fungus also releases a toxin that has been linked to laminitis. It can cause or aggravate inflammatory reactions and has a blood vessel constricting effect. A third disadvantage of grass seed hay is that the grass is sprayed to prevent disease in the seed. The grass is then sprayed to death before harvest. There is often a lot of artificial fertiliser applied and cultivation takes place on soil that has been exhausted by monoculture. Not necessarily the ideal conditions for 'healthy' hay. The fact that this hay comes from only one grass species does not benefit the horse either.

IS WILD HAY GOOD FOR MY HORSE?

Wild hay, alpine hay and eco hay are terms for hay that is obtained from natural areas. The soil in these areas has remained unfertilised for a long time, as a result of which the nutritional value, sugars and the amount of minerals in the hay that comes from it vary and are usually unknown. There is also a higher risk of the presence of unwanted and poisonous plants. On the other hand, the varied composition can also be good for your horse. You will need to have this hay tested for composition and quality.

OLD HAY HAS HARDLY ANYTHING IN IT, DOES IT? SHALL I FEED IT?

As soon as grass is cut, photosynthesis (the conversion of water and carbon dioxide into oxygen and sugars) stops. A reverse process now begins. Sugars are converted into water and carbon dioxide. This continues until the moisture content of the grass clippings drops below 40%. Grass that has been dried long enough therefore produces hay with few non-structural carbohydrates. Some people feed very old hay, thinking it contains even fewer non-structural carbohydrates. This is not the case. Old hay only contains fewer vitamins. In particular, vitamins A, D and E. Especially if your horse does not eat grass, but only hay, vitamin E is very important.

CAN I GIVE SILAGE OR HAYLAGE?

Grass preserved by fermentation is called silage. It is wrapped in plastic when the moisture content of the clippings is still over 70%. It contains a lot of proteins. Some of the proteins are broken down into ammonia. This puts a strain on the liver and kidneys and disrupts the bacterial culture in the large intestine. Not good for a horse that has laminitis or is prone to it. Haylage is grass that is packed when the moisture percentage of the clippings is between 40% and 60%. The grass has had more time to grow and therefore contains less protein than grass silage. The dry matter content of haylage is higher than that of silage grass. If you want to feed haylage, you should apply the same selection criteria as for hay: coarse-stemmed, low in non-structural carbohydrates and as high a dry matter content as possible.

IS SOAKED BEET PULP GOOD FOR FEEDING MY HORSE?

Beet pulp is left over from the production of sugar from sugar beet. The sugar is therefore no longer there. What remains are only easily digestible dietary fibres. These contain a lot of calories that are released slowly. The sugar and starch content combined is less than 8%. It is therefore a good food for horses that are laminitic or can easily become so. Because beet pulp does not contain enough vitamin A and selenium, it should not be the main part of your horse's diet. It is high in iron, which is not so good for insulin resistant horses. It can also be difficult to get the ratio of calcium to phosphorus right if you are feeding a lot of beet pulp. It is best to consult a nutritionist if you want to feed beet pulp.

I WANT TO GIVE MY HORSE A TREAT NOW AND THEN.
WHAT IS SAFE TO GIVE?

However much your horse likes apples, horse sweets, sugar cubes and other snacks, it does not need them. These snacks are even plain unhealthy for horses with laminitis. If you want to give your horse a food reward or just something to snack on, the following treats are safe for him: zucchini, pumpkin, cucumber, celery, lettuce, cabbage leaf, sunflower and pumpkin seeds, peanuts with shell and pea pods.

HOUSING AND MOVEMENT

I WANT TO CHANGE THE HOUSING FOR MY LAMINITIC. WHAT CAN I DO?

Wouldn't it be great to have 70 acres of wild land for your horse to roam all year round in a small herd? The reality is that most horse owners have limited space, time and resources to fully meet their horse's natural social, feeding and exercise needs. Do not let this stop you from looking in that direction. Your horse's environment is one that can always be improved and every step in the right direction counts. With some creativity and co-operation from others, a lot is still possible. In any case, try to keep your horse out of the stable as much as possible. Stable rest is not a solution but one of the partial causes. In a box, the horse can hardly move. This causes the blood circulation in the hooves to deteriorate. On top of this comes stress, which causes an increased production of cortisol and adrenaline. If possible, you should offer continuous turnout with a walk-in stables or natural shelter. Of course, you only do this when the grass is considered 'safe' and therefore contains as few sugars as possible (see the question 'When is grass low in carbohydrates?' on page 95). If you do not have access to pasture, put your horse in a paddock or riding arena as much as possible. If there is no paddock, you can sometimes create a temporary solution by fencing off part of the yard. If all this is really not possible, you can perhaps pull a few stables together into a bigger space. On page 107 you can read what a paddock paradise is. This is by far the best housing for your laminitic horse.

MY HORSE IS AT A YARD WHERE I CANNOT PUT HIM IN A PADDOCK AS MUCH AS I WANT. HOW DO I FIX THIS?

Is the yard manager not allowing it, do you have no time to get your horse in and out of the paddock or is it really impossible? In the first case, it is best to talk to the manager again. Explain that it is very important for now that your horse gets the opportunity to move around as much as he needs. In the second case, you could possibly make a deal with other horse owners. If you take their horses out in the morning, they can take your horse in again in the evening. Together, you can often achieve a lot. If it is really not possible for another reason, then maybe you can use the riding arena to put your horse in. Or it may be time to look for a yard where your horse can get the space it needs. Until then, get your horse exercising by hand walking him, doing ground work or games.

THE YARD MANAGER REFUSES TO FEED MY HORSE DIFFERENTLY FROM THE OTHER HORSES. WHAT SHOULD I DO?

What looks like unwillingness is often ignorance. Explain to the yard manager about sugars, hay types, soaking and beet pulp. Be patient and non-judgmental. Bear in mind that someone who has been successfully running a horse boarding business for 25 years may not be receptive to advice from someone who is 'just starting out'. Why not lend out this book for a week? Your vet could also tell them that there is a medical need for an adapted diet. Some people are more sensitive to the vet's authority than to a client's wishes.

It could also be that the yard manager understands the importance of a different diet, but just doesn't have the time to do it differently for just one horse. Offer to help or do some other task in return for the extra time they spend soaking hay for your horse. You could trade services with another boarding customer as well. They will keep the slowfeeder filled for your horses and you will take care of moving the fencing for strip grazing.

And of course, there are yard managers who think it is all just nonsense. "Horses have been fed grain for hundreds of years and it should stay that way". The solution is then: the 'H' of horse stabling, in the Yellow Pages.

WHAT IS A PADDOCK PARADISE?

Have you ever walked around in a modern zoo and admired how the living conditions of wild animals are imitated as closely as possible? With a paddock paradise, you can do the same for your horse. A paddock paradise is an environment that provides as much as possible for the natural social, nutritional and exercise needs of horses. The idea is based on the fact that in the wild, horses always follow the same fixed routes that connect watering holes, grazing areas, minerals and other interesting elements. The starting point is a wide track around the property, connected here and there to a number of larger paddocks or pieces of pasture. Along the route, you can create all kinds of natural elements and challenges to stimulate movement. For example, you can place hay feeders, water troughs and salt licks far apart from each other and build walk-in stables or natural shelters. You can integrate hedgerows or tree lines.

Different kinds of surfaces with pavers, concrete slabs, pea gravel and rocks are also common in the paddock paradise. Although, for a horse with sensitive hooves, this is not always the best choice. It can cause overloading and pain. If your horse is already living in a paddock paradise, see if you can remove these elements, replace them with rubber mats or fence them off with a safe fence.

WHEN MY HORSE IS IN THE STABLE, DO I HAVE TO INSTALL STABLE MATS?

Laminitis horses often suffer more when their feet are on hard surfaces. This is because the damaged lamellae and the sometimes inflamed sole dermis come under more pressure. As you cannot leave your horse on hoof boots 24/7, rubber mats can offer a temporary solution. Choose mats with a drainage system. Urine can then flow away via the underlying floor. This prevents fungi and bacteria and therefore reduces the risk of thrush and white line disease. You will still need to remove the mats regularly to clean the area. Let us repeat: stable mats are an emergency solution in case you really have no other solution than to lock up your horse in a stable.

SHOULD I FERTILISE THE PASTURE?

If the grass plant lacks nutrients, growth will not be good. The sugar content of the grass increases. Nitrogen and phosphorus deficiencies, in particular, cause sugar-rich grass. Grazing horses take up nitrogen through their feed. Most of it is lost in the air via the manure. If there is a shortage of nutrients in the soil, the grass also does not contain the vitamins and minerals that are important for your horse or the ratio of certain minerals is not right. In a meadow where the grass is not growing well, there is also a risk of overgrazing and therefore having grass that is high in sugar.

Fertilising can offer a solution, but don't start fiddling around with fertilisers yourself. First have a soil analysis done. This will show the state of the nutrients in the soil. With fertilising advice from the laboratory, you can then fertilise in a targeted and sensible way. The aim must be to balance the nutrients for normal growth. After all, you don't want the grass to grow like crazy because of the fertiliser. What you do want is diversity in the vegetation of your meadow. Not every fertilisation advice takes this into account. Emphasise to the laboratory that you think this is important.

If you use artificial fertiliser, your horse will have to stay somewhere else temporarily. These chemical fertilisers are toxic and can cause SIRS-related laminitis. Do not let your horse graze until the rain has removed all the fertiliser from the grass and washed it into the ground. It is best to use natural, animal-based fertilisers. The use of compost or humus is also a safe way of fertilising. However, the composition of this type of fertilisation cannot be matched to the deficiencies in the soil. This is a disadvantage.

SHALL I MOW THE MEADOW NICE AND SHORT?

You do not want flowering or seed-bearing grass in your meadow. The flowers and seed heads contain a lot of non-structural carbohydrates. Horses are known to love these and even look for them when grazing. With a good grazing plan, such as strip grazing and pasture rotation, try to prevent grass from flowering, forming seeds or becoming too short.

If mowing is the only solution to prevent flowering, do it carefully. Mowing when there are no flowers or seed heads in the grass is unnecessary and can even increase the amount of sugar in the grass. Set the cutting height so that the part of the stem containing the developing seed heads is cut off. The grass will now produce more shoots and take better root. There is no point in mowing shorter. Mowing too short even makes the grass get too much sunlight, which increases the amount of NSC. It is needless to say that the grass clippings are not horse feed.

IS IT BEST TO PUT MY HORSE IN THE FIELD AT NIGHT OR RATHER DURING THE DAY?

Between roughly midnight and 10 am, the sugar content of the grass is at its lowest. For a horse with hormonal problems that is prone to laminitis, it would be a good idea to only let it out to pasture during this period. If the temperature at night drops below five degrees, the amount of sugar in the grass increases. Therefore, grazing is not recommended during cold nights.

I HAVE A FOREST PLOT NEXT TO MY FIELD. SHALL I LET MY HORSE IN THERE?

Shadow slows down the rise of sugar content in the grass during the day. There is a lot of shade in the forest. The grass that grows there is therefore usually low in sugar. Your horse also has to make more effort to find its food among the forest plants. This slows down the rate at which it eats. The food enters the digestive tract more slowly and evenly and the carbohydrates are digested better. And then there is the extra movement that your horse gets. This is because woodland is more challenging than pasture. However, you should be aware of the presence of undesired plants and trees and obstacles such as stumps, rabbit holes or old fences. A horse with extremely sensitive hooves should not be allowed to walk on difficult ground just yet. It may be possible with solid, well-fitting hoof boots.

MY HORSE WILL HAVE TO BE KEPT ALONE FOR A WHILE. HOW CAN I MAKE SURE THAT HE DOES NOT GET BORED OR STRESSED?

A horse that is taken from its herd and set aside easily becomes upset. The stress this causes is not good for its recovery. In addition to the effect described on page 35, a solitary horse can move out of restlessness and insecurity. This puts a strain on his hooves. Make sure he can see his buddies or give him the company of one of them or a sheep or goat. Company is very important for a laminitic horse. It not only provides more exercise, but also makes the horse feel better. A horse that feels better heals better.

If company is not possible, at least make sure that he sees you often. Brush him, cuddle him, play with him and talk to him. If he is in a stable, you can hang a ball or a turnip. This does not work miracles, but some horses amuse themselves with it for a while. Fetching pieces of sour apple from a water trough is also something that some horses find amusing.

WHEN WILL MY HORSE BE ABLE TO MOVE AGAIN?

After checking with your vet, your horse can be allowed to move carefully and under supervision from Obel 1 onwards. If you are not sure whether your horse is in Obel 1 or 2, you can also watch how he reacts to movement. If he walks noticeably better after one minute, this is an indication that he can handle some movement. Let an objective outsider assess this as well. There is a risk that you are too eager for your horse to improve and are therefore asking too much of him too soon.

Let him move on properly trimmed hooves and preferably on hoof boots with soft insoles. Also, make sure that you know and have dealt with the cause of the laminitis.

WHEN CAN WE START RIDING AGAIN?

Do not ride until your horse is back at Obel 0. By the way, do not think that Obel 0 equals 'completely cured'. The amount of pain certainly does not always reflect how much the hoof tissues are still damaged. Furthermore, the horse's sole should be about 1 cm (0.4") thick. Your hoof care provider can determine this by approximation. The vet can tell with certainty from an X-ray. At the beginning, ride with hoof boots with insoles. Gradually and evenly increase the length and intensity of your rides. Do not make the distances too long, do not overload the horse and ride at a slow to moderate pace. Ride on a surface that is not too hard (asphalt) or too soft (very loose sand). Let your horse decide where he puts his hooves. Pay attention to any signs of pain or tiredness in your horse and respect them. Riding should be for his benefit, not for yours.

HOOF CARE

CAN MY HORSE BE BAREFOOT?

Of the five million years that the horse has existed, it has not been walking on its own beautiful bare feet for about five thousand. That is one thousandth of his entire existence. It would be odd if, in that short period of time, its hooves had changed so much that it would have to rely on a clothed monkey with a hammer, an anvil and some pieces of iron to walk normally. Fortunately, today we know that if living conditions and usage are adjusted in favour of the horse, any healthy horse should be able to walk on its own hooves. Whether every rider, trainer, vet, insurance company and sponsor thinks this should be the case for every horse is a question we will not answer in this book.

But what about the word 'healthy', two sentences before? Isn't there a reason why there are all kinds of modern therapeutic shoes specially developed for horses with laminitis? Indeed, there is. Whether it does what it is supposed to do is another matter. Much of it focuses on treating symptoms or is based on assumptions or outdated knowledge about anatomy, tissue function and biomechanics. Some shoes have been developed based on the results of scientific research. That research then focuses on a single aspect. Improving that one aspect does not mean that all the other disadvantages of shoeing will magically disappear. Plus, these studies hardly ever compare special shoes to hoof boots or the barefoot approach. It is fair to say that good research into the effect of corrective trimming on laminitic hooves is also scarce.

Having already adapted the horse's diet, housing, and exercise to its nature and needs, it would be a good idea to continue along these lines when it comes to hoof care. A good, modern hoof care provider knows very well how to help a laminitic without resorting to iron solutions.

WHAT IS THE BEST WAY TO TRIM A LAMINITIC HOOF?

Trimming a laminitic hoof is hardly any different from trimming a healthy one. In both cases, a modern hoof care provider focuses on balancing the hoof, improving its shape and optimising the distribution of forces. In the case of laminitis, this reduces pain, improves the hoof mechanism and thus leads to faster recovery. Simply put, the goal of trimming is to grow a healthy hoof capsule around the internal foot. Consider the hoof capsule as the shoe of the internal foot. The better this shoe fits, the better your horse moves, the faster it heals.

Because the back of the hoof is generally unaffected by laminitis, we want the horse to bear its weight there. This provides good shock absorption, good circulation and ensures that the hoof properly breaks over. A second and very important goal of trimming is to take the pressure off the damaged lamellar connection so that it can grow back into a healthy state. We also do not want pressure from the coffin bone from the inside on the sole. The latter two points require the coffin bone to be parallel to the ground when the horse loads its hoof in motion. We cannot, of course, explain in one small page how all this is done, but in general it comes down to this:

- The heels are kept low, in line with the widest part of the frog, and possibly slightly bevelled. Your hoof care provider tries to promote heel first landing this way. Also, the coffin bone will come parallel to the ground in this way.
- The pressure in the quarters (sides) of the hoof is taken off to improve the health of the hoof cartilages (collateral cartilages).
- The hoof wall in the toe area is trimmed and rounded off to keep it off the ground and to minimise stress on the damaged lamellar connection. If necessary, the lamellar wedge (see p. 25) is partially rasped away.
- Flares are removed as they generate excessive stress to the lamellar connection.
- Normal sole tissue remains untouched because all healthy sole provides valuable cushioning.

- The bars are trimmed to reduce pressure on sensitive tissues in the hoof.
- The frog retains its function as a shock absorber and carries a considerable part of the weight. Where it blocks the collateral grooves, your hoof care provider will trim it back. Dirt must be able to get out of the grooves.
- Parts of the frog and white line that are affected by bacteria or fungi are cut clean and treated.

HOW OFTEN SHOULD MY HORSE BE TRIMMED?

Laminitic hooves need to be trimmed much more frequently than those of a healthy horse. In the beginning, your hoof care provider will be on your doorstep every three weeks. Later, that may be cut down to every five weeks. In between visits, you may need to pick up a hoof rasp to do some maintenance yourself. Your hoof care provider will explain to you exactly what to do and what not to do.

As long as the shape and balance of the hoof are not restored, the force acting on the damaged tissues in the hoof will perpetuate the problem. Your hoof care provider will want to remedy this as quickly as possible. That is why they suggest visiting so often. The remedy should not be worse than the disease. Lowering high heels, for example, is not something to be done in one go, but rather in stages. That way too much tension on the deep flexor tendon can be prevented. Also, the hoof can be so deformed that the blood flow is pinched off. Certain amino acids that are important for hoof growth do not get to the right places in the hoof at the same time. This causes your horse to have cup-shaped hooves with high heels. Frequent trimming helps to solve this problem.

It is expensive to have your hoof care provider come so often, but you get what you pay for. Skimping on hoof care will slow down the healing process considerably. In the end, you might end up with vet bills that are much higher than those of your hoof care provider.

WHAT IS THE DIFFERENCE BETWEEN NATURAL, PHYSIOLOGICAL AND TRADITIONAL TRIMMING?

There are many names for different methods of trimming. The most fanatical proponents of each method claim that the other camp is destroying the horse's feet. Traditional farriers are accused of always trimming each and every hoof as if it will be shod and then not shoeing it. Their response is that they always have to put up with the misery of the natural trimmers who have taken only a weekend course. The physiological trimmers fight each other over the height of the heels or whether or not to trim the frog. If you like drama, you should definitely go along with it.

If you are more results-orientated, then you look at the knowledge, skill and experience of the person trimming your horse's hooves. Do they keep up with developments in their field? Do they really understand how a hoof is anatomically and functionally put together? Are the hooves getting better and better since they have been trimming your horse? Can they explain what they are doing and why? If you have answered 'yes' four times, you may have found the right person for your horse. What kind of trimmer they call themselves is not so important.

IS A TRIMMER SOMETHING ELSE THAN A FARRIER?

Trimmer, farrier, and even equine podiatrist; these are all names for people who are professionally involved with the hooves of horses, and they are all colleagues too. As soon as someone touches a horse's feet with a pair of nippers, a rasp and a hoof knife, he or she is a hoof care provider. So, this is the broadest term. If it involves shoeing, then you are dealing with a farrier. The shoes can be made of iron or synthetic material, and the farrier can try to imitate bare feet with them. Since this book is based on unshod hooves, we use the name 'hoof care provider' for all these professionals, as long as they do not nail or glue objects to the hooves. Hoof boots thus fall under the barefoot approach. After using them, you can take them off and put them away.

HOW DO I FIND A GOOD HOOF CARE PROVIDER?

Trust comes on foot and leaves on horseback, as the saying goes. Good hoof care providers often have years of experience. That is not to say that professionals who are just starting out cannot be good, but in the case of severe laminitis you would do well to choose someone who has successfully treated more cases of this condition. That trust in their work is also reflected in the large number of satisfied clients they have. Ask around about other people's experiences with them. Someone who does a truly good job will be recommended to you from all sides. And just because your best friend says that her farrier is very nice, always on time, not too expensive and very good with horses, is no guarantee that he knows the ins and outs of laminitic hooves.

If you have found someone, don't feel obliged to ask them in advance how they deal with laminitis. If you know the main outlines of how to trim a laminitic hoof and this hoof care provider comes up with a completely different story, then ask them how that is. Don't dismiss them straight away, but let them explain why they do it the way they do. Reflect on their explanation and ask other people's opinions. Also ask if you can have a look at the hooves of other customers' horses. Of course, the customer in question should be willing to let you do so. The opinions of regional vets with whom this hoof care provider has worked may also be useful.

MY HORSE IS IN TOO MUCH PAIN TO LIFT A FOOT WHEN TRIMMED. WHAT DO I DO?

Trimming a laminitic hoof requires more time and more attention to detail than is the case with a healthy hoof. A horse that is restlessly moving back and forth does not make work any easier. If it is too painful for your horse to lift one front leg, a hoof boot on the other front leg can help. A gardening knee mat, a piece of insulation board or a bit of straw to stand on can also make a difference.

You can ask your vet for a mild sedative you can give. In some cases, even that will not be enough. The vet will then have to be there when you have an appointment with the hoof care provider to give your horse an anaesthetic injection. An additional advantage is that these two professionals can then exchange views on your horse's condition. If your horse is in so much pain, it may be even better off in a veterinary clinic. Ask your vet how they see this.

MY HORSE IS SENSITIVE OR EVEN LAME AFTER THE TRIM. IS THAT NORMAL?

Many things are not right in a laminitic hoof. After a trim, the load on both diseased and healthy tissue is different. Your horse may have to get used to this or may just have to get through it. It may even cause him to be sensitive for a while. A good hoof care provider will see this coming and warn you about it. They will also explain what is causing the sensitivity and how long they expect it to last. The best thing, of course, would be if your horse did not have any sensitivity at all. Your hoof care provider can advise you on the use of hoof boots to take care of this.

Your horse should not be really lame after a trimming. If it is, the trim has been too drastic or too careful. Lowering very high heels all at once is asking for trouble. Not trimming the bars sufficiently, so that they pinch the soft tissues inside the hoof, can also cause pain. The lameness may be caused by the farrier's ignorance, lack of insight or experience. Very unpleasant, but certainly something you should discuss with them. You are not going to tell them how to work, but you can say that you don't think it is right for your horse to be lame after every trim. Don't be fobbed off with an answer like, "Who is the professional here?" A real professional does not trim a horse lame.

Let's be honest. It could be indirectly caused by you. Sometimes your hoof care provider needs X-rays to make the right assessment. If they ask for them and you don't have them taken, you might ask yourself whose fault it is that your horse doesn't walk as good as it should following the trim.

Your hoof care provider has had to work more or less at a guess. Follow their advice carefully and consistently. Not going to ride means not going to ride. If you get on your horse anyway, then you can't blame others if things go wrong.

WHAT CAN I DO MYSELF BETWEEN TRIMMING APPOINTMENTS?

Trimming a laminitic hoof requires experience, insight, knowledge and skill that very few horse owners have. This is because it is usually the first time that they have had to deal with such a hoof. That is why you leave it to a professional hoof care provider. Even if you trim your other horses' hooves yourself. In close consultation with your hoof care provider however, you can still do useful work in between their visits. They can explain how to keep the toes of the hoof short so that they do not touch the ground. That way, there is no pressure on the damaged lamellar connection, which speeds up the healing process. The same applies to flares (see p. 26). Complications such as a frog infection or white line disease (p. 120) should be treated daily. You can do that after your hoof care provider has cut the area clean and started the treatment. They will tell you which products to use.

Never cut or rasp a laminitic hoof on your own, it's for the best. You will do more harm than good before you know it. Ask your hoof care provider if there is anything you can do and, more importantly, how you can do it. Let them also judge your work.

MY HORSE NOW HAS A HOOF ABSCESS. IS THAT NORMAL? WHAT SHOULD I DO ABOUT IT?

If the blood circulation in the hoof is reduced, for example due to a build-up of fluid (oedema), dead tissue and accumulated blood are not drained off properly. It becomes infected and causes a hoof abscess. Abscesses of this kind appear one to two months after the onset of laminitis on the coronary band, in the white line or above the heel bulbs.

In case of a coffin bone rotation or a sinker, the coffin bone presses against the sole from the inside. This causes tissue to die off. In addition, a sole bruise can occur. With a bruise, the quality of the horn of the sole decreases. Bacteria can penetrate and cause a sole abscess. The risk is even greater in thin soles. Bacteria can also enter the hoof via the stretched white line or the lamellar wedge.

Abscesses are a medical problem. They must be dealt with by the vet. Unfortunately, farriers have become accustomed to this task. Their tools are not sterile, and they cannot provide the follow-up care that is needed. If things go wrong, you end up with new abscesses, an infection or even blood poisoning.

After the vet has opened an abscess, you can take care of it by keeping the wound clean and bandaging it. The vet will explain to you how this is done. The hole made in the hoof wall by a coronary band abscess breaking out will grow downwards. Keep an eye on that spot. It is possible that a fungus will settle there. If so, treat with an antifungal agent. Often, ordinary kitchen vinegar with a few drops of tea tree oil will do.

In order to prevent cutting, you can wait until the abscess matures and breaks out on its own. To speed up this process, some people soak the hoof in warm water with soap. Although this is effective, be aware that it weakens the sole and the white line. It increases the chance of new bacteria penetrating.

WHAT IS WHITE LINE DISEASE?
SHOULD I TREAT IT MYSELF?

White line disease is a deterioration of the hoof wall caused by a combination of bacteria and fungi. This infection can only occur if the horn quality of the hoof wall is already of moderate quality. The bacteria and fungi are therefore not the main cause. It is a job for your hoof care provider to treat white line disease. Often, a large part of the hoof wall has to be removed. After that, you need to treat the affected area regularly. There are all kinds of products for this. Your hoof care provider or vet will decide on the best remedy depending on how severe the damage is. You should not just pick something yourself. The stronger the substance, the greater the chance of dehydration and damage to healthy or growing tissue.

Prevention is always better than cure. Try to find out why the quality of the horny tissue is so bad. This can often be traced back to nutrition. Deficiencies in certain trace elements and amino acids, as well as wrong proportions of iron, copper, zinc and manganese are associated with poor horn tissue. Mechanical causes, such as an excessively long hoof wall or stance abnormalities that overload the hoof wall, also cause damage that gives fungi access. The deformed hoof wall in the case of laminitis is also a well-known cause. Substances in the horse's dung and urine attack the horn cells. Hooves that are too wet make the sole and white line too soft, while hooves that are too dry tear easily. The fungus benefits directly from this. Hoof nail holes are also often the start of white line disease.

DOES MY HORSE NEED HOOF BOOTS?

Yes, we would like to see all horses barefoot all the time. No, using hoof boots does not change that. Boots are an aid to help horses get through the time it takes to heal better, faster and pain-free. After some time, you will no longer need them. Pain-free movement ensures better blood circulation and faster development of all the tissues in the hoof. Through adequate movement, oedema disappears more quickly. Hoof abscesses are less common in horses that have boots. Let's also not forget that movement burns sugars and therefore stimulates weight loss. Movement also increases sensitivity to insulin.

With hoof boots, your horse can be used again more quickly. The faster recovery can help boost your motivation. Your horse will only benefit from this. Boots can finally get some horses out of the cycle of being laminitic, healing and getting laminitis again. It will not be the first time that a horse has escaped euthanasia thanks to a pair of boots.

Another great thing about boots is that they can be taken off after use. This allows the hooves to be trimmed regularly. The hoof care provider or boot fitter can use all kinds of insoles to provide optimal protection and shock absorption for your horse's painful hooves. The sole of the shoe can be cut and rasped in order to perfectly position the break over point.

WHICH BOOTS DOES IT NEED THEN?

The time when you could only choose from two brands and three models is fortunately a thing of the past. There are many types of boots. Some brands make special therapeutic boots. These are not made for riding, but are ideal for the first period of recovery. Other boots can be adapted in all sorts of ways. There are boots for normal or very intensive use. There are expensive boots and relatively cheap ones. So, there is no simple answer to this question. A good hoof care provider or a specialised boot fitter can advise you on which boot is best for your horse. Also ask about the experiences of others. There are facebook pages and websites entirely dedicated to this topic.

HOW DO I FIND THE RIGHT SIZE OF HOOF BOOT?

Ill-fitting hoof boots are difficult to put on, irritate the coronary band, heel bulbs and bulb groove and come off when you ride. So, buy boots that fit well. Before you can do this, you need to measure the size. You do this on a correctly trimmed hoof. The hoof should not have been trimmed more than a fortnight ago. The measurements are based on the length and the widest part of the hoof. The length is the distance between the toe and the back of the heel. So do not measure up to the back of the heel bulbs. The widest part of the hoof is exactly half way down the hoof, between the tip of the frog (apex) on one side and the end of the bars and the central groove of the frog on the other (see image on the next page). You might also want to ask your hoof care provider. They have experience with measuring hooves.

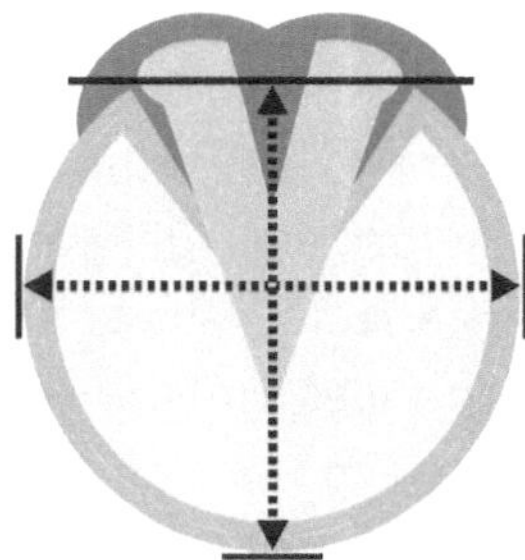

Sizes usually have some overlap. If the length and width of your horse's hooves fall into different sizes, it is best to choose the larger of the two. If the difference is more than one size, see if another model or brand of shoe has a size that fits your horse's hooves. There are even hoof boot fitters nowadays.

In the case of laminitis, there is also the fact that the shape of the hoof can change quite considerably. Boots that are fitted at the moment that the white line has stretched significantly will probably no longer fit as the hoof heals. Good news for your horse; not so good for your wallet. This should not be an obstacle. You can keep the costs down with second-hand boots. Just make sure that they are not worn at an angle.

CAN HOOF BOOTS STAY ON 24/7?

Hoof boots are not made to be worn around the clock. If you want to try this anyway, make sure you choose lightweight boots. They should fit perfectly and should certainly not rub. Water should be able to drain off easily. Protect the coronary band and heel bulbs with bandages, socks or a bit of Vaseline, if necessary.

Nowadays, there is a kind of hoof protection that is a cross between hoof boots and glue-on shoes. It is, as it were, a hoof boot that is glued on. The disadvantage is that you cannot trim the hoofs regularly, the advantage is that they offer protection 24/7. Your hoof care provider or boot fitter can tell you more about this.

WHY ARE HOOF BOOTS SO EXPENSIVE COMPARED TO HORSESHOES?

The reason why boots are expensive is that the production process is a lot more complicated than with horseshoes. Different materials are used and everything has to fit together perfectly. Although shoes are expensive, they are still more economical than shoes. Horseshoes wear out with every step your horse makes whereas you take boots off after use. This makes them last much longer. A lot of boots are also made in such a way that you can replace the different parts.

WHAT KIND OF THERAPEUTIC SHOEING IS OUT THERE?
DOES IT HELP?

Often therapeutic shoeing is used to treat laminitis. The range of corrective shoes for laminitic horses varies from open-toed shoes or even reversed shoes to shoes resembling an unshod natural hoof, from egg bar shoes to shoes with adjustable heel height and synthetic glue on shoes. The shoes are attached with or without all kinds of insoles and shock absorbing materials. Some shoes include frog support (heart bar shoes), or even a screw mechanism that can be used to increase or decrease the pressure on the frog.

We have already mentioned that this kind of shoeing often focuses on combating symptoms. It is true that some shoes can have a positive effect on an anatomical part of the hoof or on a biomechanical function of a tissue. This does not mean, however, that all the disadvantages of shoeing then suddenly no longer exist. There are, in fact, many disadvantages to the use of metal footwear. The hoof mechanism cannot function optimally, whereas this is so important for the healing of laminitis. A second major problem is that all the force that the hoof exerts on the ground is transmitted via the shoe to the lamellar connection. This is precisely the damaged tissue that is unable to absorb this force. This is what we call peripheral loading.

The following is a short list of the disadvantages of shoeing:
- In between shoeing appointments, the hoof wall cannot be maintained with a rasp or knife. The outer wall can quickly become too long and will then start pulling on the lamellar connection like a lever.
- Because the sole of a shod hoof is lifted off the ground, it will not harden sufficiently. A solid sole will provide more protection to the coffin bone that is pushing against it from the inside.
- Sole flexibility reduces when hooves are shod, increasing the chance of sole bruising.
- A heart bar shoe puts continuous pressure on the digital cushion. The latter needs alternating pressure and pressure relief to stay in good health.
- Shoes with raised heels are used to reduce the tension of the deep digital flexor tendon, but increase the pressure on the tip of the coffin bone and the lamellar connection at the front of the hoof. In addition, the deep flexor muscle tension will adjust to the new position. This causes the forces exerted by the tendon to return to the old level quite quickly. Raising the heels is a temporary solution that unfortunately is often applied for too long.
- Shod horses cannot feel the surface they walk on. They stumble more often and occasionally slip. For laminitic horses this is very painful and may result in less movement than is beneficial.

If you still want to use shoes despite all the disadvantages mentioned above, choose plastic over metal and glue rather than nails.

I AM TERRIFIED OF REMOVING THE SHOES FROM UNDER MY HORSE. SHOULD I REALLY DO THIS?

It seems strange to take the shoes off a horse when it is laminitic. You may feel that you are removing the last bit of protection. Yet you are doing the right thing. Remember that the sensitivity that can occur is caused by years of shoeing in combination with the laminitis, not by the removal of the shoes themselves. The blood circulation has been poor all that time and the quality of the tissues in the hoof has suffered greatly as a result. The sole and the frog are not well developed and are therefore sensitive. If the horse has been put on shoes too young, the digital cushion and hoof cartilages are poorly developed. Once again, the magic word: hoof boots. If you had painful feet, would you rather wear shoes with soft, springy rubber soles or clog around on metal shoes? It is no different for your horse. For the times when he does not have his shoes on, make sure that the ground is soft. Have the shoes removed by a hoof care provider. This is also the person who will now trim the hooves in a way that will lead as quickly as possible to recovery.

WHAT IF MY HORSE REALLY CAN'T DO WITHOUT?

A horse that is said to be really unable to do without shoes usually has serious hormonal problems, severe damage to the tissues of the internal foot or both. Neither of these problems can be solved with a piece of iron. In almost all other cases, it has an owner who is unable or unwilling to provide the conditions necessary for good, healthy bare feet. Unfortunately, these owners seldom look for the blame in themselves. If the farrier then says that the horse is better off with a metal prosthesis, the horse can say goodbye to barefoot recovery.

WHAT ARE SYNTHETIC SHOES?
IS IT BETTER THAN REGULAR SHOES, BAREFOOT OR HOOF BOOTS?

The order of what is good for your horse's hooves is: barefoot, boots, synthetic shoes, traditional metal shoes. Synthetic shoes can be made entirely of synthetic material or have a metal core. The first is better than the second. If it is glued, it is better than if it is nailed. Synthetic shoes have some of the disadvantages that metal shoes also have, although sometimes to a lesser extent. A few of these disadvantages also apply to hoof boots. There is the force of inertia (which one can feel in a car that suddenly takes a sharp bend) that acts on bones, joints and capillaries. However, most movement and exercise during the recovery period of laminitis will be in walk. The inertia force will not be too great then. Peripheral loading occurs, as mentioned on page 124. With synthetic shoes, the horse does not feel the ground well and can therefore stumble more often. Regular rasping of the hoof to keep the toe short and the heels low is also out of the question. Horseshoes, no matter what material, increase the length of the toe and thus the leverage on the painful lamellar connection. Furthermore, it is quite a hassle for the farrier to apply glue on shoes. The hoof must be spotless, completely dry, and not too cold. But let's just say that is the farrier's problem.

I HAVE PUT PHOTOS OF MY HORSE'S HOOVES ON FACEBOOK. NOW I AM GETTING CONTRADICTORY ADVICE. HOW SHOULD I DEAL WITH THIS?

Just to be sure, read again the answer to the question 'Who should I believe?' on page 85. Conflicting advice is almost always given with the best of intentions. The point is that you should not rely on advice based on two or three pictures taken with your phone. To start with, it is not easy to take pictures of hooves that give a good idea of the state of the hoof. What looks skewed in a photo can be perfectly straight in real life and vice versa. Furthermore, it is difficult to give all the information that is necessary for proper advice. The web experts tumble over each other with questions and especially comments under your post and you will hardly have the time to answer everything. This almost never stops anyone from making a judgment. Among the people who give advice are people with years of experience and people who hardly know a thing. You just don't know who is who. Nobody sees the horse in the flesh or has the opportunity to hold and examine the hoof.

Of course, two people see more than one. Maybe the advice will help you look at the hoof differently. That is good. But if you have questions or doubts about your horse's hooves, discuss them with your hoof care provider or one of their colleagues in the first place. Taking a course yourself is also a good idea. You will learn a lot about how hooves should be and how trimming works. That makes it easier to talk to your hoof care provider and to separate the wheat from the chaff on Facebook advice.

AND WHAT ABOUT ME?

HOW DO I COMMUNICATE WITH THE VETERINARIAN
AND THE HOOF CARE PROVIDER?

Here is a cliché: the vet has a high status. Their word is law. They spent years of study and have cured hundreds of horses with laminitis. Therefore, they do not need your opinion. Another killer: the farrier is a grumpy guy who you can't get any angrier than telling him how to do his job. The reality is that these types exist, but hopefully not around your horse. Good vets and hoof care providers listen carefully to their clients. You see your horse every day, know its idiosyncrasies and its usual behaviour and deviations. You see things they do not.

Now for the answer to the question. Open up a conversation. Do this in person or by telephone. Written communication can easily be misread and you cannot clarify or adjust anything. Be clear, but also friendly and respectful in your communication. Prepare the conversation. Write down your questions in advance. Tell what your expectations are and ask whether they are feasible. Listen carefully to the answers and write these down as well. If you don't understand the answer, say so. Don't fall into the trap of 'yes but'. It is better to say: "You say that my horse is doing much better, but I do not see the improvement. Are we both perhaps overlooking something?" Also remember that you are looking at your horse from a completely different point of view. They have a professional view, while you have a strong emotional bond with your horse. It doesn't hurt to remind each other of that from time to time. Also tell them when you get too much information. It takes time to process new information. Professionals sometimes forget that. Summarise the conversation at the end by saying: "So if I understood correctly, we are on the right track. I just need to pay more attention to how I exercise my horse". In this way, you give the other party the opportunity to check whether his message has come across well.

MY VET AND MY HOOF CARE PROVIDER DISAGREE.
WHAT SHOULD I DO?

The answer to this question follows on from the previous one. You will have to enter into a conversation, only this time with two people. Maybe they are more in agreement than you initially think. You can find out by just talking to them. Suggest to each what the other thinks about it and ask for a reaction. Even better is if they discuss it with each other, preferably with you present. They may have different ideas about what your expectations are. If you speak to them together, you can explain things. Of course, it is also possible that they are diametrically opposed to each other. One swears by therapeutic shoeing with silicone soles; the other would rather see them removed today than tomorrow. Now it is starting to look like an unmanageable situation, but it can still work out. When you have decided which approach is the most compatible with what you want, here's what you can do. Ask the other person if they see possibilities and are willing to continue the treatment with the solution you have chosen. Maybe this solution is not their preference, but they still might want to continue. If this is not the case, there is only one option: thank them for their services so far and look for someone to complete your team of caregivers. Explain to the new practitioner what happened and ask them beforehand if they agree with the path you have chosen. This will prevent further disappointment and delay in the healing process.

I HAVE MY DOUBTS ABOUT THE WORK OF MY HOOF CARE PROVIDER.
WHAT IS THE BEST APPROACH?

It gets almost boring to say it again, but you should discuss your doubts with them. Maybe they have a good reason for trimming differently than you expect. Make sure you know what you are talking about. The answer to the question 'What is the best way to trim a laminitic hoof?' on page 114 is a good starting point, but no more than that.

Be concrete and personal in your communication. You won't make friends if you say: "On Facebook, they say you take too much off the frog". Put your doubts to them in a question form. For example, ask: "I see that you trim the frog quite short. May I ask why? Because I can imagine that my horse needs a large frog now that his feet are so sensitive". This sounds less confrontational. Listen carefully to the answer and see if it makes sense to you. In this example, it may be that the hoof care provider is opening up the collateral grooves at the back to allow any dirt to get out. This looks radical, but it is not. Moreover, it is necessary.

Feel free to ask another question. But be careful not to dwell on it. If you are about to say, "And yet I think the frog is much too short", then perhaps you should consult another hoof care provider. This may also be the time when you start sharing your doubts. Tell them that you are going to do so. Tell them as well you are going to take photos of the hooves to show in a Facebook group or to another hoof care provider. Also reassure them that you will not mention their name. It's tempting to do so, but it's not important right now.

If you are satisfied, you can tell them that too. Even the worlds grumpiest farrier likes to hear that their customers are happy with them. You'll see that it makes them go that extra mile for you and your horse. It really does.

I HAVE MY DOUBTS ABOUT WHAT MY VET SAYS.
WHAT DO I DO?

It is no different with the veterinarian than with the hoof care provider. The difference is that - barring exceptions - vets are more highly trained, have less time to spare for a client, and are less used to having assertive clients. Don't worry, just use the same method. You are the customer, and your horse's health is at stake. If you don't feel comfortable expressing your doubts, ask someone else to be there when you do so. Believe it or not, some vets speak differently in front of a yard manager they have known for 20 years than they do in front of a 16-year-old girl with her laminitic Shetland pony.

HOW DO I ASSESS OBJECTIVELY HOW MY HORSE IS DOING?

Looking at your horse in a neutral way is almost impossible. Your emotional bond is getting in the way and you really want him to get better. Yet it is important that you learn to look objectively. Fluctuations in his condition, which always occur, will then not immediately rob you of hope. The numbers tell the tale, we say. The circumference of the neck can be measured and noted (see p. 52), as can fever and pulse. You can estimate his weight weekly (p. 63) and write it down. Put this kind of data into a table and you will soon see which way things are going. If you are handy with Excel, you can conjure up graphs that give you even more insight.

Lameness is more difficult for you as a layperson to determine. What you can do is give a daily lameness score on a scale of 1 to 10. Even if you think it is too positive or too negative, you can see the big picture. Ask someone else to do this for you. Preferably, it should be someone who doesn't know your horse very well. Your hoof care provider will probably also want to tell you what they see each time they trim and whether they think if there is progress or not. You can also keep a sort of journal of this. If your horse has a relapse, it is easier to see the big picture if your hoof care provider said before and after that it was going well.

Take clear photos of your horse's hooves, front, side, back and bottom. Save them in a folder on your computer and create subfolders with the date you took the photos. If you find that the hooves are not improving after six months of trimming, it can be a big surprise to see the photos from six months ago.

A comprehensive questionnaire that you can fill in together with your hoof care provider or your vet to find out as much information as possible about your horse is available for free download here:

understandinglaminitis.com/product/laminitis-the-horse-owners-checklist-for-cure-and-prevention/

I WANT SO MUCH TO DO SOMETHING FOR MY HORSE, BUT WHAT?

The fact that you have almost finished this book shows that you are indeed very motivated to help your horse. You are doing all you can to address the causes. You are paying close attention to nutrition, housing, exercise and hoof care. You have probably found experts who can help you with this. It is now up to you to guide their efforts with your horse. Watch out for the pitfall of 'two captains on one ship'. If different people treating your horse give you contradictory advice, this will certainly not speed up the healing process. It is your horse; you decide what happens. Make sure that everyone who is involved in the recovery of your horse is on the same wavelength. Ask critical questions. Make clear communication agreements and set goals. Make sure that everyone knows what the expectations are. Growing old pain-free is not the same as returning to advanced level dressage. Also make sure that you don't become rigid. Try to improve the circumstances and the treatment for your horse. Observe carefully to see what the result is. Adjust your chosen strategy if necessary.

WHERE DO I FIND SUPPORT?

Caring for a laminitic horse is time-consuming, expensive and emotionally draining. Even if you have the time and the financial resources to provide proper care, the emotional aspect is still something you have to deal with. It is difficult to see your horse in pain. The hoped-for recovery can take a long time or not come at all. Your friends at the stable go out riding every day, while you are soaking hay and are happy if your horse makes a few careful steps. Sometimes, the people around you don't understand this at all. They don't see what it means to you and may even make hurtful comments such as, "Gee, it's only a horse. I would take him to the butcher". It is very important for you and therefore for your horse that you feel good and strong during this difficult period.

The solution is simple: find people who do understand you. These can be other horse owners who have had the same experience. But people who have not had to deal with it themselves can still be a great source of support. They have seen their horse struggle with a different disease, or their dog, their cat or even their goldfish. There are many horse groups on Facebook. There are large groups with a general focus, smaller groups specifically for certain breeds and also special groups on laminitis or PPID. You are bound to find buddies here who will be happy to support you. Hang in there, you are doing great!

WHERE DO I FIND MORE INFORMATION ABOUT LAMINITIS?

In the facebook groups we talked about in the previous answer, you can find a lot of information. Please read page 85 again before you do. If you are still hungry for knowledge about laminitis, order the book 'Laminitis: understanding, cure, prevention'. 266 pages, full-colour, with all the ins and outs and the latest scientific insights. You can order it here:

understandinglaminitis.com/order/

New articles appear regularly on understandinglaminitis.com and on facebook.com/understandinglaminitis

www.ingramcontent.com/pod-product-compliance
Lightning Source LLC
Chambersburg PA
CBHW022141150726
47992CB00002B/698